PSYCHIATRIC EMERGENCIES

Essential Strategies for Rapid Assessment and Effective Intervention

Dr. William Rudduck
MBBS, FRANZCP
Consultant Psychiatrist

Copyright © 2024 Dr. William Rudduck
All rights reserved.

No part of this publication, Psychiatric Emergencies: Essential Strategies for Rapid Assessment and Effective Intervention, may be reproduced, distributed, or transmitted in any form or by any means, including photocopying, recording, or other electronic or mechanical methods, without the prior written permission of the author, except in the case of brief quotations for educational or review purposes.

Acknowledgements

The journey of creating Psychiatric Emergencies: Essential Strategies for Rapid Assessment and Effective Intervention has been both rewarding and enlightening, and I owe its completion to the invaluable support and inspiration of many individuals.

I extend my deepest gratitude to my mentors and colleagues, whose wisdom and expertise have significantly shaped my understanding of acute psychiatric care. Your guidance and encouragement have been instrumental throughout this process.

To the healthcare professionals I have had the privilege to work alongside, your dedication to patient care and resilience in challenging situations are the foundation of this book. I am particularly indebted to those who shared their insights and experiences, enriching the practical perspectives presented here.

To my family and friends, your unwavering support and belief in this endeavor have been my constant source of strength.

Finally, I would like to thank the patients who have entrusted me with their care. Your courage and stories have provided the inspiration to make this book a meaningful contribution to the field of mental health.

This book is a testament to the collective effort of those committed to improving psychiatric emergency care.

Dr. William Rudduck
MBBS, FRANZCP
Consultant Psychiatrist
2024

Preface

Emergencies in psychiatric care demand not only a deep understanding of mental health but also the ability to act decisively, efficiently, and with empathy. Psychiatric Emergencies: Essential Strategies for Rapid Assessment and Effective Intervention serves as a comprehensive guide for mental health practitioners, emergency department personnel, and students navigating the complexities of acute psychiatric care.

This book was inspired by years of frontline clinical experience managing crises in psychiatric settings. The challenges faced by healthcare professionals during these critical moments, coupled with the need for evidence-based approaches, underscored the importance of a resource that combines practical insights with current research. The field of psychiatric emergencies is rapidly evolving, and this book seeks to bridge the gap between theory and practice, offering actionable strategies for clinicians across diverse settings.

The text is structured to provide a logical flow, beginning with foundational concepts of psychiatric emergencies and progressing to advanced interventions tailored to specific conditions. Topics such as rapid assessment protocols, pharmacological interventions, de-escalation techniques, and care coordination are presented in detail, with a focus on their application in real-world scenarios. Each chapter is enriched with case studies, illustrative examples, and clear algorithms to aid decision-making.

Special attention is given to the management of agitation, violence, and acute behavioral disturbances—areas often fraught with complexity and urgency. Drawing from robust evidence and clinical guidelines, this book equips professionals with the tools necessary to ensure patient safety, staff well-being, and optimal outcomes.

The intended audience for this work includes psychiatrists, emergency medicine specialists, nurses, and other allied health professionals involved in psychiatric care. Students and trainees will also find this text invaluable as they develop the skills and knowledge needed for effective practice in high-pressure environments.

It is my hope that this book will serve not only as a practical resource but also as a source of inspiration for those committed to advancing the field of mental health. As we continue to confront the complexities of psychiatric care, may this guide empower us to approach each crisis with confidence, compassion, and resilience.

Dr. William Rudduck

MBBS, FRANZCP
Consultant Psychiatrist
2024

Acknowledgement
Preface
Table of contents

Table of Contents

Chapter 1: Understanding Psychiatric Emergencies

1. Introduction
   - The Growing Demand in Emergency Departments (EDs)
   - Importance of Initial Assessment

2. Critical Risks in Psychiatric Emergencies
   - Suicide and Self-Harm
   - Violent Behavior and Potential for Assault
   - Risk of Absconding

3. Differentiating Organic Illnesses and Substance Use

- Recognizing Organic Mimics of Psychiatric Conditions
- Impact of Substance Use on Psychiatric Presentations

4. Epidemiology of Mental Health Disorders
    - Burden of Mental Health Disorders Globally and in Australia
    - Trends in Emergency Department Presentations
    - Factors Contributing to Increased ED Visits

5. Mental State Examination in the ED
    - Addressing Knowledge Gaps and Education Needs
    - Bias, Stigma, and Discrimination in Healthcare

6. Conducting the Mental Health Assessment
    - Immediate Risk Identification

- Key Components of Assessment: Appearance, Behavior, and Communication

7. Mental Health Triage and Risk Management
    - Mental Health Triage Scale and Risk Stratification
    - Managing High-Risk Patients

8. The Formal Psychiatric Interview
    - Key Components: Demographics, Presenting Complaint, Mood, and Affect
    - Thought Processes and Content Assessment
    - Insight, Judgment, and Observation

9. Comprehensive Assessment of Mental Health Disorders
    - Evaluating Psychotic Symptoms and Thought Content
    - Assessing Perception, Cognitive Function, and Physical Examination

10. Emerging Models of Care in Mental Health
    - Specialized Mental Health Teams in EDs
    - Challenges and Solutions in Emergency Psychiatry

11. Conclusion
    - Importance of Timely and Collaborative Assessment
    - Future Directions in Emergency Psychiatry Management

Chapter 2: Differentiating Medical and Psychiatric Causes of Mental Health Symptoms

1. Introduction
    - Challenges in Identifying Causes of Mental Disorders

- Classification of Causes: Psychiatric, Medical, Intoxication-Related, and Behavioral
- The Role of the Diagnostic and Statistical Manual of Mental Disorders

2. Key Concepts
    - Reducing Morbidity and Healthcare Costs
    - Importance of Comprehensive Evaluation
    - Identifying Substance-Related Disorders
    - Recognizing Delirium and Cognitive Deficits

3. General Approach
    - Medical Clearance in Emergency Departments (EDs)
    - The Importance of Comprehensive History and Examination
    - Challenges in Differentiating Medical and Psychiatric Causes

4. Factors Influencing Diagnosis
    - Indicators of Organic Causes (Medical):
    - Abnormal Vital Signs
    - Delirium and Cognitive Impairments
    - Neurological Deficits
    - Abrupt Onset of Symptoms
    - Indicators of Psychiatric Causes:
    - Psychiatric and Family History
    - Slow Onset and Gradual Deterioration
    - Hallucinations and Personality Changes

5. Diagnostic Framework for Emergency Physicians
    - A Simple DSM-V-Based Classification for Mental Disorders
    - Role of Triage in Identifying High-Risk Patients
    - Safety Considerations in Patient Management

6. The Interview Environment
    - Creating a Safe and Private Setting

- Building Trust During Psychiatric Interviews

7. History-Taking and Collateral Information
    - Identifying Contributing Medical and Psychiatric Factors
    - Substance Use and Medication Compliance
    - Family History and Risk Assessments

8. Physical Examination
    - Importance of Thorough Neurological and Systemic Evaluation
    - Recognizing Signs of Endocrine and Metabolic Disorders

9. Emerging Trends and Challenges
    - Integration of Community-Based Psychiatric Services
    - Addressing Emergency Department Pressures
    - Managing Substance-Related Disorders

10. Differentiating Between Medical and Psychiatric Conditions
    - Limitations of Medical Clearance in EDs
    - Comprehensive Assessment Techniques

11. Conclusion
    - The Necessity of Thorough Evaluations
    - Innovations in Models of Care

Chapter 3: Defibrillate Self-Harm and Suicide

1. Introduction
    - Definition of Suicide and Deliberate Self-Harm (DSH)
    - Significance in Emergency Medicine
    - Challenges in Identifying and Assessing At-Risk Individuals

2. Epidemiology
    - Global and Regional Statistics

- Trends in Suicide and DSH
- Age, Gender, and Sociocultural Disparities

3. Risk Factors for Suicide
    - Static and Dynamic Risk Factors
    - Psychiatric and Medical Influences
    - Impact of Social and Cultural Factors

4. Repeated Episodes of Deliberate Self-Harm
    - Characteristics of High-Risk Individuals
    - Predictors of Repeat DSH
    - Chronic Suicidal Ideation and Co-Morbidities

5. Frequent Emergency Department Attendances
    - Association with Suicide Risk
    - Key Indicators for Further Intervention

6. Aetiology of Suicide and DSH

- Psychological, Social, and Medical Contributors
- Role of Acute Psychological Distress

7. Triage and Initial Management
    - Resuscitation and Stabilization
    - Mental Health Triage Protocols
    - Safety Measures in the Emergency Department

8. Suicide Risk Assessment
    - Principles and Frameworks
    - Collateral Information Gathering
    - Limitations of Current Risk Assessment Tools

9. Management Strategies
    - Multidisciplinary Approach
    - Immediate and Long-Term Interventions
    - Patient-Centered Care and Collaboration

10. Risk Stratification and Disposition

- Inpatient vs. Outpatient Care
- Criteria for Psychiatric Admission
- Follow-Up and Community Support

11. Legal and Ethical Considerations
    - Local and Regional Frameworks
    - Balancing Safety and Autonomy

12. Conclusion
    - Key Takeaways for Clinicians
    - Opportunities for Early Intervention
    - Enhancing Outcomes through Integrated Care

Chapter 4: Depression Management and Intervention Strategies

1. Introduction
    - Importance of Depression Assessment in the ED
    - Differentiating Clinical Depression from Mood Fluctuations

2. Epidemiology
    - Prevalence and Recurrence
    - Gender Differences and Age of Onset
    - Long-term Impact of Depression

3. Aetiology
    - Genetic and Environmental Factors
    - Neurobiology of Depression
    - Precipitating Life Events

4. Prevention
    - Public Health Initiatives
    - Role of Emergency Department Staff

5. Clinical Features
    - Symptoms and Severity Indicators
    - Impact on Daily Functioning
    - Onset and Progression of Depression

6. Signs and Features of Depression: Detailed Analysis
    - Psychomotor Agitation vs. Retardation
    - Affective State and Thought Content
    - Level of Insight

7. Variants of Depression
    - Melancholic Depression
    - Psychotic Depression
    - Mild and Moderate Depressive Episodes

8. Special Populations
    - Depression in the Elderly
    - Brief Depressive Reactions
    - Grief and Depression

9. Differential Diagnosis
    - Bipolar Depression vs. Unipolar Depression
    - Organic Mood Disorders

10. Diagnostic Considerations
    - Assessing Comorbidities and Functional Impairment
    - Psychosocial Context in Diagnosis

11. Chronic Dysthymia
    - Characteristics and Prevalence

- Exacerbation into Major Depression

12. Anxiety Disorders and Depression
    - Overlap and Differentiation
    - Co-occurrence of Anxiety and Depression

13. Personality Disorders and Depression
    - Risk Factors and Comorbidities

Chapter 5: Psychosis

1. Key Points
    - Emergency Department as a Crucial Assessment Site
    - Differentiating Psychosis from Organic Causes
    - Risks Associated with Acute Psychosis
    - Collaborative Treatment Planning

2. Introduction
    - Psychotic Disorders and ED Presentations

- Challenges in Managing Psychotic Patients in the ED
- Engaging Family Members and Caregivers

3. Classification of Psychotic Disorders
    - Ruling Out Medical Causes
    - Substance Use Evaluation
    - Provisional Psychiatric Diagnosis
    - Psychological Stress Assessment

4. Epidemiology and Prognosis
    - Schizophrenia and Bipolar Disorder Prevalence and Course
    - Suicide Risk and Recovery Patterns

5. Aetiology and Prevention
    - Genetic and Environmental Factors
    - Secondary Prevention Strategies

6. Clinical Features
    - Delirium and Dementia
    - Psychosis with Clear Consciousness
    - Medication-Induced Psychosis

7. Psychotic Symptoms and Related Syndromes
   - Manic Syndrome in Bipolar Disorder
   - Mixed Affective Psychosis
   - Delirium Versus Mania
   - Mania Versus Acute Schizophrenia
   - Psychotic Depression
   - Substance-Induced Psychosis
   - Reactive Psychotic-Like States

8. Assessment of Psychotic Patients
   - Key Questions in Assessment
   - Mental State and Risk Evaluation

9. Initial Stabilization and Management
   - Engaging the Patient
   - Mental State Examination
   - ORisk Assessment

10. Comprehensive Medical and Psychiatric Evaluation
    - Medical Evaluation and Investigation

- Collaborative Discussion Between Physicians and Psychiatrists
- Diagnostic Investigations

11. Chronic Psychotic Illness and Comorbidities
    - Associated Physical Health Issues in Chronic Psychotic Disorders

12. Emergency Department Management
    - Psychiatric Diagnoses in the ED
    - Behavioral and Pharmacological Interventions
    - Management of Drug-Induced Psychosis, Acute Schizophrenia, and Mania

Chapter 6: Pharmacological Approaches to Managing Patient Agitation

1. Introduction
    - Managing Agitation in the Emergency Department (ED)
    - Patient Assessment Before Sedation

- Importance of Patient Safety and Communication

2. General Principles of Rapid Tranquilization
    - First-Line Medications: Benzodiazepines and Antipsychotics
    - Oral vs. Intravenous Administration
    - Importance of Medication Familiarity
    - Desired Outcomes and Patient Monitoring
    - Environmental Considerations for Sedated Patients
    - Supportive Care and Patient Privacy

3. Risks of Rapid Tranquilization
    - Over-sedation and Respiratory Depression
    - Cardiac Risks: QT Prolongation and Sudden Cardiac Death
    - Hypotension and Dystonic Reactions
    - Neuroleptic Malignant Syndrome (NMS) and Anticholinergic Effects

- Seizure Risk and Delirium in Repeated Dosing
- Special Considerations for Elderly Patients

4. Pharmacological Agents
    - Benzodiazepines
    - Midazolam: Rapid Onset and Risks
    - Diazepam: Prolonged Half-Life and Respiratory Depression
    - Clonazepam: Long-Term Sedation and Risks of Accumulation
    - Lorazepam: Balanced Sedation with Fewer Side Effects
    - Antipsychotics
    - Droperidol: Potent Sedation with Cardiac Considerations
    - Haloperidol: Long-Acting with Risk of Extrapyramidal Effects
    - Olanzapine: Atypical Antipsychotic with Lower Extrapyramidal Effects
    - Risperidone: Effective with Postural Hypotension Risk

5. Patient Selection and Dose Adjustments
   - Adjusting Medication for Elderly and Medically Complex Patients
   - Individualizing Treatment Based on Medical History and Risk Factors

6. Conclusion
   - Safeguarding Patient and Staff Well-being
   - Ongoing Monitoring and Re-assessment of Treatment Efficacy

Chapter 1
Understanding Psychiatric Emergencies

This chapter addresses the growing number of patients presenting to emergency departments (EDs) with mental health concerns. It highlights the necessity of conducting an initial assessment promptly upon the patient's arrival, focusing on critical risks such as:

Suicide and self-harm

Violent behavior or potential for assault

Risk of absconding

The chapter also emphasizes the importance of distinguishing organic illnesses that may mimic psychiatric conditions. Additionally, it examines the increasing role of substance use or misuse as a contributing factor in psychiatric presentations to EDs, underscoring the need for comprehensive and efficient evaluation.

Epidemiology of Mental Health Disorders

Mental health disorders rank among the top three contributors to the overall burden of disease and injury in Australia, alongside cancer and cardiovascular disease. They are leading contributors to non-fatal disease burden, with approximately 4 million Australians experiencing a common mental disorder in 2015. The impact of mental illness is profound, carrying significant human and socioeconomic costs.

Major depressive disorder, for instance, is as debilitating as conditions like congestive heart failure or chronic severe asthma. Its prevalence is expected to rise sharply in the coming decade. Suicide, a critical public health concern, is the third leading cause of death among Australian men across all age groups, with rates of 16 per 100,000 men and 5 per 100,000 women. The risk is particularly high in men aged over 85, with rates reaching 37.6 per 100,000. A significant proportion of those who die by suicide have had contact with healthcare providers, often within emergency departments (EDs), in the preceding year.

Between 2006 and 2014, ED visits in the United States increased by 14.8%, while mental health-related presentations rose by 44%, contributing to ED overcrowding. A similar trend has been observed in Australia. Factors contributing to this surge include:

Limited access to private health insurance

Rising substance abuse

Insufficient social support and housing

Lack of alternative care options

The 24/7 availability of ED services

According to the Australian Institute of Health and Welfare, mental health-related ED visits numbered 276,954 in 2016–17. This accounts for nearly 4% of public hospital ED presentations, consistent with international estimates of 2–6%. However, these figures likely underestimate the true scope, as many individuals present with concurrent medical issues that mask underlying mental health conditions.

Patients aged 15–44 represent two-thirds of these presentations, with anxiety, substance abuse, mood disorders, and schizophrenia or delusional disorders being the most common diagnoses. Approximately 17.7% of hospitalized adults report a mental health issue within the past year, and 0.4–0.7% of adults experience psychosis annually. These statistics underscore the importance of mental health awareness in emergency medicine, as mental illness often remains undiagnosed or unrecorded in hospital data systems.

Mental State Examination in the ED

Knowledge Gaps and Education Needs

Emergency department clinicians often report challenges in managing mental health presentations due to gaps in knowledge and experience. Australian studies highlight deficiencies in risk assessment skills, particularly regarding self-harm, aggression, and distinguishing psychiatric from medical conditions. Many clinicians express a need for enhanced education on mental health-related cases.

Substance use often complicates mental health assessments, leading to prolonged ED stays and delayed dispositions. Furthermore, mental health patients may be triaged into lower urgency categories and experience longer wait times compared to other patients, highlighting systemic biases. Efforts are underway to improve care quality and patient experience for individuals presenting with mental health issues.

Addressing Bias, Stigma, and Discrimination

Patients with mental illnesses frequently face discrimination and barriers to accessing care. Healthcare providers must recognize how their own biases and values might affect assessments. When negative attitudes are identified, seeking guidance from a senior colleague is advisable.

Conducting the Mental Health Assessment

The mental health assessment begins with identifying immediate risks, such as:

Suicide

Violence or aggression

Absconding

A triage nurse and treating physician should gather collateral history from family, carers, or emergency services and devise a preliminary treatment plan. This ensures the safety of the patient, staff, and others while maintaining dignity and respect throughout the process.

Key components of the assessment include:

Appearance, behavior, and communication

Risk evaluation for self-harm, aggression, substance use, and neglect

Information from community-based resources, such as general practitioners, is incorporated to develop a provisional diagnosis and management plan. Disposition is coordinated with mental health services to streamline care delivery.

Mental Health Triage and Risk Management

The Mental Health Triage Scale, integrated with the Australian Triage Scale (ATS), assists in categorizing patients based on risk and urgency. Categories include:

ATS 2: Imminent danger, requiring police escort or restraint

ATS 3: Acute psychosis or distress with potential aggression

ATS 4–5: Chronic mental health issues requiring less urgent care

Risk factors for dangerous behaviors—such as aggression, intoxication, or prior absconding—are systematically assessed using tools that stratify patients into high, medium, or low risk.

For high-risk patients, EDs may deploy specialized teams, including mental health clinicians and security personnel, to respond in a coordinated manner. Sedation or restraint is used only as a last resort, in accordance with legal and institutional guidelines.

Goals of Mental Health Assessment

The primary objectives of mental health evaluations in the ED are:

1. Identifying the presence of a mental illness.

2. Assessing immediate risks to the patient or others.

3. Determining the appropriate setting for treatment—community-based care or hospitalization.

The Formal Psychiatric Interview

Introduction

A comprehensive psychiatric assessment relies on two fundamental components: the patient's history and the mental state examination (MSE).

Gathering a thorough history involves collecting relevant details about the patient's current presentation to the emergency department (ED). This process enables clinicians to understand the nature, duration, and severity of symptoms, as well as the events triggering the ED visit. Effective history-taking combines keen observation, active listening, and empathetic communication to establish rapport and foster a collaborative treatment approach.

An MSE is constructed alongside the history to facilitate the identification of potential diagnoses and risks. During the initial moments of the interview, clinicians should aim to pinpoint key problems and themes, directing subsequent questioning to delve deeper into potential diagnostic considerations.

Environmental Considerations

The environment in which an MSE is conducted is critical. Patients in behavioral distress often feel fearful and overwhelmed, especially in the high-stimulation setting of an ED. To mitigate these challenges:

The interview space should be quiet and private to create a sense of safety.

Clinicians should minimize interruptions and ideally sit at the same level as the patient unless risk factors dictate otherwise.

Respect, empathy, and genuine communication should be emphasized, with a calm and nonjudgmental tone to help de-escalate heightened emotions.

For safety, clinicians should be aware of exit routes, ensure the availability of duress alarms, and involve security personnel if risks are anticipated. Patients may be searched for dangerous items, such as weapons or medications, according to institutional policies.

Key Elements of the Psychiatric Interview

1. Demographic Information

The initial part of the interview involves collecting basic demographic data. These details provide essential context for follow-up care and help build a profile of the patient's lifestyle, relationships, and support systems. Topics may include:

Residential history

Occupation and employment history

Household composition

Social resources (family, friends, and partners)

Knowledge of previous medical and psychiatric hospitalizations, including treatment types and follow-up arrangements, is also critical for tailoring care.

2. Presenting Complaint

Patients are asked to recount the sequence of events leading to their ED presentation. This exploration focuses on:

Circumstances surrounding the behavior

Degree of planning or impulsivity

Involvement of substances (e.g., drugs, alcohol)

Understanding the patient's recent experiences (e.g., isolation, bereavement, or health crises) and usual coping mechanisms provides insight into their current difficulties.

3. Mood and Affect

Clinicians assess the patient's mood (internal emotional state) and affect (external expression of mood), noting any inconsistencies, rapid mood swings, or incongruences.

Subjective mood descriptions (e.g., "sad" or "angry") can be supplemented with a numeric rating scale.

Objective indicators include appetite, sleep patterns, hygiene, and ability to concentrate.

Direct questioning about thoughts of self-harm or suicide is vital. A clear and detailed plan for suicide necessitates immediate intervention.

4. Thought Processes and Content

Assessment of thought processes involves examining the coherence, organization, and fluency of the patient's ideas. Common thought disorders include:

Circumstantiality: Long-winded explanations eventually reaching the point.

Tangentiality: Irrelevant responses that fail to address the question.

Flight of Ideas: Rapid, fragmented thoughts that are difficult to express coherently.

Thought content focuses on identifying delusions or hallucinations, which may indicate psychotic disorders. Delusions (e.g., persecutory or grandiose beliefs) and hallucinations (e.g., auditory or visual) should be explored in detail, including their context and impact on the patient's functioning.

5. Insight and Judgment

Insight reflects the patient's understanding of their condition, ranging from denial of illness to full awareness and acceptance of treatment needs. Evaluating insight and judgment helps determine the appropriateness of treatment strategies and the likelihood of adherence.

Observation During the Interview

1. Appearance, Attitude, and Behavior

Clinicians should observe the patient's physical presentation, behavior, and attitude. Key factors include:

Grooming and hygiene

Eye contact (e.g., avoidance or intense staring)

Unusual or repetitive behaviors (e.g., rocking or hand-wringing)

Speech characteristics (e.g., rate, volume, tone, and rhythm)

Restlessness, aggression, or agitation may necessitate early de-escalation measures.

2. Speech and Communication

Speech patterns offer critical clues to the patient's mental state. Abnormalities may include:

Mute: Total absence of speech.

Poverty of Speech: Slow or monosyllabic responses.

Pressure of Speech: Extremely rapid and loud speech.

Fluency, logical coherence, and appropriateness should also be evaluated.

Comprehensive Assessment of Mental Health Disorders: A Structured Overview

Psychotic Symptoms: Characteristics and Assessment

Psychosis often manifests through disorganized and incoherent speech, characterized by illogical progression and a lack of clear connections between ideas. This can range from milder forms such as circumstantiality to more severe disruptions like derailment or word salad. These speech patterns differ based on the underlying condition: flight of ideas is commonly observed in mania, whereas poverty of thought or thought blocking may indicate schizophrenia or catatonia.

Evaluating Thought Content

A mental health evaluation includes analyzing the patient's recurring themes or concerns. Common themes include hopelessness, helplessness, suicidal ideation, grief, loss, or feelings of persecution. Patients may also express delusions, including:

Religious or grandiose delusions: Exaggerated self-importance or divine association.

Delusions of poverty or nihilism: Beliefs that parts of the self or the world do not exist, are decaying, or are dead.

Assessing Perception

Auditory hallucinations are the most prevalent form of hallucinations in psychiatric disorders. Patients may actively hallucinate even while denying it during questioning. Subtle indicators, such as unexplained shifts in gaze or apparent attentiveness to unheard voices, may reveal ongoing auditory hallucinations. These observations are critical in detecting command hallucinations, which may prompt harmful actions.

Cognitive and Physical Examination

Assessing cognitive function and conducting a physical examination are fundamental to psychiatric evaluation. This ensures that behavioral abnormalities are not caused by an acute medical condition, such as delirium. Key aspects of cognitive evaluation include orientation, concentration, attention, memory, language, and abstract reasoning. Impairments in these areas influence diagnosis, treatment planning, and patient disposition.

Notably, approximately 20% of mental health patients present with concurrent medical conditions that require attention. Diagnostic investigations may include:

Blood tests (e.g., electrolytes, liver/renal function, CK levels).

Thyroid function evaluation.

Drug toxicology screening.

Imaging (e.g., CT scans).

Lumbar puncture, as indicated by clinical findings.

The Importance of Timely Assessment and Collaboration

A thorough mental health evaluation facilitates accurate diagnosis and enables tailored treatment plans. Emergency department (ED) personnel must collaborate with mental health professionals to ensure seamless transitions to specialized care when necessary. This approach minimizes delays, reduces risk, and enhances outcomes.

Emerging Models of Care in Mental Health

The role of specialized mental health teams in EDs is evolving. Trends include the establishment of dedicated psychiatric short-stay units within or adjacent to EDs. While these models improve patient access to specialized care, they may inadvertently de-skill ED personnel. Nevertheless, the presence of mental health professionals promotes knowledge sharing and enhances interdisciplinary capacity.

Challenges in Emergency Psychiatry

Despite advances, mental health patients often face access blocks and prolonged ED stays due to bed shortages. These delays risk suboptimal care and over-reliance on sedation or restraint practices. Addressing these systemic issues requires collaboration between ED and mental health teams to develop solutions that prioritize patient safety and dignity.

Conclusion

Effective mental health assessment and management in emergency settings are pivotal to addressing the growing demand for psychiatric services. By adopting structured assessment protocols and fostering interdisciplinary collaboration, healthcare providers can ensure timely, high-quality care for mental health patients.

References

1. Meadows G., Grigg M., Farhall J., et al. Mental Health in Australia: Collaborative Community Practice. Oxford: Oxford University Press; 2012.

2. Australian Institute of Health and Welfare. Australian Burden of Disease Study: Impact and Causes of Illness and Death in Australia 2011. Updated May 2016.

3. Moore B., Stocks C., Owens P. Trends in Emergency Department Visits, 2006–2014. HCUP Statistical Brief #227; 2017.

4. ACEP Clinical Policies Subcommittee. Clinical Policy: Critical Issues in the Diagnosis and Management of the Adult Psychiatric Patient in the Emergency Department. Ann Emerg Med. 2006;47:79–99.

5. Shea S. Psychiatric Interviewing. 3rd ed. Elsevier; Philadelphia.

[Full reference list available upon request].

Chapter 2
Differentiating Medical and Psychiatric Causes of Mental Health Symptoms

Key Points:

1. Reducing Morbidity and Costs: Differentiating between medical and psychiatric causes of mental health issues in emergency department presentations helps decrease both morbidity and healthcare costs.

2. Comprehensive Inquiry: Always assess whether there is an underlying medical condition in addition to psychiatric symptoms to identify potential medical causes of mental disorders.

3. Importance of Thorough Examination: Missed diagnoses often result from failing to

conduct a detailed medical history, mental state evaluation, and physical examination.

4. Identifying Substance-Related Disorders: These disorders are most easily detected through direct patient history or collateral information from others.

5. Delirium and Cognitive Deficits: The presence of delirium or new cognitive impairments strongly suggests an underlying organic or substance-related condition.

6. Repeated Evaluation for Delirium: Accurate diagnosis of delirium may require multiple assessments over time to fully evaluate the condition.

Introduction

Emergency physicians (EPs) often encounter patients presenting with suspected mental disorders. The primary challenge is to identify the underlying cause of the disorder. These causes can be broadly classified into psychiatric, medical, intoxication-related, and behavioral categories. Accurate identification of the cause, alongside careful consideration of the capabilities of local medical facilities, leads to appropriate patient management, reducing both morbidity and healthcare costs.

EPs require a simple classification system that aligns with the Diagnostic and Statistical Manual of Mental Disorders, 5th edition (DSM-V), helping to communicate diagnoses clearly with psychiatric colleagues. Such a system facilitates accurate diagnosis, management, and disposition. Table 20.2.1 outlines a proposed classification framework for emergency settings.

While the term "organic" has traditionally referred to medical causes of mental disorders, there is growing recognition of potential medical bases for certain psychiatric conditions. The concept of "medical clearance" has been in practice for over four decades, yet there is no universal agreement on its exact definition or required procedures. At its core, medical clearance seeks to identify medical conditions that may either cause, aggravate, or coexist with mental disorders, directing patients to appropriate care. However, this process is viewed as an imperfect strategy to reduce risks.

General Approach

Patients presenting with abnormal behavior that is initially attributed to psychiatric conditions often have an underlying medical cause. Studies indicate that the incidence of medical conditions contributing to mental disorders ranges from 19% to 80%. Differentiating between medical and psychiatric causes is often challenging, as there are few clear-cut indicators that can easily distinguish the two. Comprehensive patient history, physical examination, and mental state assessments are essential to reach a differential diagnosis.

In some cases, the diagnosis can be made quickly after taking a thorough medical and psychiatric history, alongside a mental status and physical examination. Other cases may require more extensive investigations, repeated assessments, and close monitoring to reach a final diagnosis.

Medical clearance in emergency departments (EDs) can be unreliable, especially in cases involving intoxication or other factors that hinder proper assessment. A non-judgmental approach, combined with prudent interventions based on known risks, careful monitoring, and repeated assessments, often yields the most accurate diagnosis and the best clinical outcomes.

Studies have shown that ED staff and psychiatrists frequently miss medical conditions when performing medical clearance. This oversight is commonly due to factors such as inadequate history-taking, failure to seek collateral information, neglecting physical examinations (including vital signs), and uncritical acceptance of medical clearance by psychiatric teams. Failure to reevaluate the patient's condition over time also contributes to missed diagnoses. The most successful identification of medical conditions often comes from the triage nurse or medical officer, who asks whether any medical conditions exist in addition to the psychiatric complaints.

Classification of Mental Disorders for Emergency Physicians

A simple classification of mental disorders based on DSM-V terminology helps emergency physicians differentiate between psychiatric and medical causes of mental illness, ensuring appropriate management and disposition. The classification includes various categories, such as delirium, dementia, substance-related disorders, and other psychiatric conditions.

Triage and Safety Considerations

Triage plays a crucial role in identifying patients who may have underlying medical conditions contributing to their psychiatric presentation. Proper identification by nursing staff reduces morbidity and mortality. Many psychiatric patients may pose a significant risk to themselves or others and require urgent intervention. Safety-related questions should always be addressed to ensure the patient's and staff's safety.

A triage checklist can help nursing staff identify high-risk patients, ensuring that those with a potential organic illness receive the necessary medical evaluation in the ED. In some cases, patients with known psychiatric conditions and low medical risk can be referred directly for psychiatric evaluation, bypassing the medical clearance process. These decisions are based on consensus guidelines developed by emergency physicians and psychiatrists.

In cases where a psychiatric diagnosis is likely, the appropriate urgency rating according to the Australasian Triage Scale should be applied. This system categorizes psychiatric presentations based on urgency, ensuring that patients are seen within appropriate timeframes.

The Interview Environment

The environment in which a psychiatric interview takes place is essential for obtaining accurate information. A quiet, private setting is ideal, although safety concerns may limit the choice of location in emergency situations. Establishing trust with the patient is key, as many details shared during the interview can be sensitive.

History-Taking

A thorough medical history is crucial in identifying medical conditions that may contribute to a mental disorder. Substance use, including compliance with prescribed medications and use of recreational or over-the-counter drugs, should be thoroughly explored. Gradual onset and a previous psychiatric history often suggest a psychiatric origin, while abrupt onset without prior psychiatric history favors a medical cause.

Family history is an important factor in identifying the potential medical or psychiatric origins of a condition. For example, a family history of Huntington's disease or porphyria may suggest an organic cause, while a strong family history of bipolar disorder may indicate a psychiatric cause. Risk assessments for suicidal and homicidal behavior should always be part of the evaluation process to ensure patient safety.

In modern clinical practice, HIV-related illnesses have emerged as significant mimics of both psychiatric and medical conditions. Patients with a positive HIV status should be carefully assessed for any medical causes of behavioral disturbances. These conditions often present initially with mild anxiety or depression but can be treated once diagnosed.

Delirium, characterized by fluctuating levels of consciousness and attention, is another medical condition that must be considered in patients with altered mental states. It often presents abruptly and may be accompanied by changes in the sleep-wake cycle and poor recent memory. Identifying delirium is critical, as it frequently signals an underlying medical or substance-induced disorder.

Collateral History

Collateral history—information obtained from family members, caregivers, or other sources—is essential when the patient cannot provide complete or accurate information. It can clarify the diagnosis, especially in cases where the patient's mental status fluctuates. Family members may also provide important details about the patient's medical history, including medication use and previous psychiatric diagnoses.

Physical Examination

Thorough physical examination is vital to identify signs of underlying medical conditions. This includes assessing neurological status, recognizing signs of endocrine diseases, identifying toxidromes, and checking vital signs. Failure to address these areas of examination often leads to missed diagnoses, which could be life-threatening.

In clinical practice, it is crucial to distinguish whether a patient's symptoms arise from a medical or psychiatric condition. Several factors influence the likelihood of a psychiatric or organic (medical) cause being the primary diagnosis. Understanding these factors can aid in accurate diagnosis and management.

Factors Suggesting Organic Causes (Medical Illness):

Vital Signs: Abnormal vital signs are often indicative of an underlying medical issue.

Age: A first episode of psychosis in patients older than 40 may point to a medical etiology, such as neurodegenerative diseases.

Delirium: Delirium, often marked by fluctuating consciousness and impaired cognition, suggests an organic cause.

Memory Impairment: Significant memory loss and cognitive dysfunction may be associated with medical conditions like dementia or metabolic disturbances.

Neurological Signs: Symptoms like dysarthria (difficulty speaking) or other neurological deficits suggest a medical issue.

Abrupt Onset: A sudden change in behavior or mental state, occurring within hours or days, often points to an organic cause, such as an infection or a neurological disorder.

Recent Medical Issues: A history of a recent medical problem, such as a stroke or severe infection, can contribute to psychotic-like symptoms.

Medication and Substance Use: Medication side effects, drug use, or withdrawal can provoke symptoms that mimic psychiatric disorders.

Factors Suggesting Psychiatric Causes:

Psychiatric History: A past history of psychiatric illness or a family history of psychiatric disorders increases the likelihood of a psychiatric diagnosis.

Cognition: If the patient has intact cognitive function, it is more likely the issue is psychiatric in origin.

Slow Onset: Psychiatric disorders, especially chronic ones, tend to develop slowly over time, leading to gradual changes in behavior and functioning.

Premorbid Functioning: A history of slow deterioration in social, occupational, or familial aspects points towards a psychiatric condition, particularly mood or personality disorders.

Hallucinations: Visual, auditory, or tactile hallucinations, especially with specific patterns (e.g., voices arguing or commenting), are more typical of psychiatric conditions like schizophrenia.

Personality Changes: Sudden and marked personality shifts may signal a psychiatric illness, especially in the context of conditions like mood or personality disorders.

Differentiating Between Medical and Psychiatric Conditions:

Medical Clearance: The practice of "medically clearing" a patient, typically performed in emergency departments (ED), is a critical but imprecise step. The more accurate approach is to state that no acute medical issues were found that would preclude psychiatric care and further evaluation.

Comprehensive Assessment: An effective assessment includes obtaining a detailed medical and psychiatric history, performing a thorough physical and mental state examination, and conducting targeted investigations. Omitting any of these steps could lead to misdiagnosis or incorrect disposition.

Emerging Trends and Challenges:

Community-Based Psychiatric Services: An increasing number of psychiatric services are being delivered in the community, avoiding the need for hospitalization or ED involvement. However, outcomes for these models remain under-researched.

Emergency Department Pressures: The introduction of targets like the National Emergency Access Target (NEAT) has increased pressure on EDs and psychiatric services to act quickly. Despite these targets, many services struggle to meet the demands for timely psychiatric assessments and care.

Substance-Related Disorders: Patients with substance-related issues pose significant challenges. Intoxication may last for extended periods, and proper management often requires medical intervention or brief admission. EDs are experimenting with short-stay units that combine psychiatric, emergency, and substance-related care to better manage these patients.

Conclusion: The assessment of patients with suspected psychiatric illness must be thorough, incorporating both medical and psychiatric evaluations. Accurate diagnosis is vital to ensure the appropriate course of treatment and disposition, preventing mismanagement. Given the increasing demand on EDs and psychiatric services, new models of care, such as community-based management and integrated service units, are being explored to provide timely and effective interventions.

References

1. Hoffman, R. S. (1982). Diagnostic errors in the evaluation of behavioral disorders. Journal of the American Medical Association, 248, 964–967.

2. Anderson, E. L., Nordstrom, K., Wilson, M. P., et al. (2017). American Association for Emergency Psychiatry Task Force on

Medical Clearance of Adults Part I: Introduction, review, and evidence-based guidelines. Western Journal of Emergency Medicine, 18(2), 235–242.

3. Tintinalli, J. E., Peacock, F. W., Wright, M. A. (1994). Emergency medical evaluation of psychiatric patients. Annals of Emergency Medicine, 23, 859–862.

4. Olshaker, J. S., Browne, B., Jerrard, D. A., et al. (1997). Medical clearance and screening of psychiatric patients in the emergency department. Academic Emergency Medicine, 4, 124–128.

5. Pollard, C. (1994). Psychiatry Reference Book – Nursing Staff. Hobart: Department of Emergency Medicine, Royal Hobart Hospital.

6. Gert, W., Osser, D. (2009). Massachusetts Emergency Physician and Psychiatry Task Force: Community-based

medical screening guidelines for individuals with psychiatric symptoms and low medical risk. Available from: https://www.acep.org/globalassets/uploads/uploaded-files/acep/advocacy/state-issues/psychiatric-hold-issues/ma-medical-clearance-guidelines-toxic-screen-ma.pdf

7. Smart, D., Pollard, C., Walpole, B. (1999). Mental health triage in emergency medicine. Australian & New Zealand Journal of Psychiatry, 33, 57–66.

8. Folstein, M. F., Folstein, S. E., McHugh, P. R. (1975). 'Mini Mental State': A practical method for grading the cognitive state of patients for the clinician. Journal of Psychiatric Research, 12, 189–198.

9. Shah, S. J., Fiorito, M., McNamara, R. M. (2010). A screening tool to medically clear psychiatric patients in the emergency department. Journal of Emergency Medicine, 43(5), 871–875.

10. O'Sullivan, D., Brady, N., Manning, E., et al. (2018). Validation of the 6-Item Cognitive Impairment Test and the 4AT test for combined delirium and dementia screening in older emergency department attendees. Age and Ageing, 47(1), 61–68.

Chapter 3
Defibrillate Self - Harm and Suicide

Key Points

1. Deliberate self-harm is a common emergency department presentation, stemming from a range of biological, social, and psychological issues.

2. Patients who self-harm are diverse, with the majority not exhibiting ongoing suicidal behavior.

3. Suicide risk assessment post-self-harm aims to inform treatment, identify modifiable risks, and recognize protective factors. It involves evaluating demographic, psychiatric, medical, and psychosocial factors, along with the current crisis, ensuring the patient feels heard and understood.

4. No single "gold standard" exists for suicide risk assessment; risk levels can fluctuate rapidly.

5. Key predictors for repeat self-harm include psychiatric conditions, personality disorders, substance abuse, previous attempts, hopelessness, social isolation, and intoxication.

6. A structured approach should address triage, restraint, observation, medical and suicide assessments, treatment, disposition, and follow-up.

7. Effective management requires collaboration among emergency, mental health, and primary care professionals, along with family involvement.

8. Treatment decisions should be collaborative, factoring in any advance

statements and involving next of kin for additional information and cooperation.

9. The legal framework governing practice in the relevant jurisdiction should always be considered.

Introduction

Suicide is the intentional act of taking one's own life, representing the most severe form of deliberate self-harm (DSH). The spectrum of DSH can range from minor injuries to life-threatening acts. Although suicide remains relatively rare, about 10% of individuals who die by suicide visit the emergency department (ED) in the month leading up to their death, with many not receiving a psychosocial evaluation. This highlights a critical opportunity for timely intervention. Despite varied presentations, approximately 8% of ED patients have experienced suicidal ideation or behavior, though these are often not disclosed unless actively investigated. The primary challenge for emergency clinicians lies in identifying and assessing individuals at risk for suicide, with a focus on managing co-morbidities and modifiable risk factors.

DSH may reflect maladaptive coping strategies in response to psychological distress, and while not always indicative of suicidal intent, it does suggest an elevated risk for future suicide attempts. DSH is a frequent reason for ED visits, accounting for around 0.4% of all ED presentations. Management goals include addressing physical health issues, assessing the likelihood of repeated self-harm, and treating potentially reversible psychosocial factors that contribute to the behavior.

Epidemiology

In Australia, 3,128 deaths occurred due to intentional self-harm in 2017, with a higher rate in males (19.1 per 100,000) compared to females (6.2 per 100,000). Suicide accounted for 1.9% of all deaths, and, with a median age at death of 44.5 years, intentional self-harm was responsible for the highest number of Years of Potential Life Lost (YPLL), outpacing other causes such as ischemic heart disease. Globally, the suicide rate is lowest in countries such as South Africa, Greece, Mexico, Israel, and Brazil, whereas Lithuania, Hungary, Japan, and Latvia report the highest rates. The World Health Organization (WHO) estimates that low- and middle-income countries account for 78% of all suicides.

Hospital visits for DSH are significantly more frequent than suicide completions, with DSH hospitalizations being at least 10 times higher. The 2007 Australian National Survey of Mental Health indicated that approximately 1.9% of males and 2.7% of females experienced suicidal ideation within a 12-month period, with some populations exhibiting rates as high as 25%.

Risk Factors for Suicide

A history of DSH is a significant predictor of future suicide attempts, with 1% to 2% of individuals who engage in DSH completing suicide within the year following the attempt. Approximately 40% of suicides have a prior history of self-harm. A systematic review found that the suicide rate was 2% within one year and 7% after nine years for individuals with a history of self-harm. While hospitalization and aftercare can reduce short-term suicide risk, they have limited impact on long-term risk, possibly due to inadequate treatment of underlying psychiatric conditions.

Repeated Episodes of DSH

Individuals who repeatedly engage in DSH may initially receive social and medical support, particularly in younger patients. However, this is less common in patients over 60 years old. The risk of repeat DSH is significant, ranging from 12% to 16% in the year following the initial attempt, with 10% of these occurrences happening within the first week. Female patients, particularly those who are unemployed, have personality disorders (especially cluster B traits), or struggle with substance abuse, are at higher risk. Chronic suicidal ideation, multiple DSH attempts, and underlying psychiatric conditions (such as personality or psychotic disorders) increase the likelihood of eventual suicide. Identifying and addressing modifiable factors, such as substance abuse or psychological distress, is critical in preventing further episodes.

Patient Characteristics

Age: Suicide and DSH are rare in children under 12 years. Data from Australia indicate higher rates in males aged 30 to 34 (27.5

per 100,000) and females aged 50 to 54 (10.4 per 100,000), with rates rising in the elderly, particularly from age 65 onward. DSH peaks during adolescence and young adulthood (ages 15 to 24) but decreases with age.

Gender: In Australia, the male-to-female suicide ratio was 3.4 in 2010, and 2.7 in New Zealand. The incidence of male DSH has increased in recent years, with females typically selecting less lethal methods and being more likely to seek medical attention following DSH.

Social and Cultural Factors: Suicide rates are higher in individuals who live alone or are socially disadvantaged, particularly in urban areas with overcrowding and poverty. Being single, separated, divorced, or widowed increases suicide risk two- to threefold in high-income countries. Suicide rates are also notably higher among Indigenous populations, with Australian

Aboriginal and Torres Strait Islander suicide rates in 2017 being more than double that of the general population. Rural and remote areas, as well as those in prison, report higher suicide rates.

Medical and Psychiatric Factors: Chronic health conditions and untreated psychiatric disorders, including mood disorders, significantly elevate the risk of suicide. Mood disorders, especially when coupled with borderline personality disorder or substance abuse, pose the highest risk. A history of self-harm, substance misuse, or psychotic disorders, as well as ongoing mental health challenges, strongly correlate with repeated DSH attempts and eventual suicide.

Frequent ED Attendances

Individuals who frequently visit the ED (more than three times per year) have a sevenfold increased risk of suicide compared to the general population. This risk is particularly elevated among those with panic attacks and depression. A history of frequent ED visits should prompt further evaluation and intervention to reduce long-term suicide risk.

Aetiology of Suicide and DSH

Suicide and DSH are often precipitated by personal crises, life changes, or poor social support, compounded by psychiatric conditions or substance use. Alcohol or drug intoxication may lower inhibitions and increase the likelihood of suicidal acts. Research has shown that a significant portion of individuals who attempt DSH have considered the act for less than 10 minutes, underscoring the role of acute psychological distress in precipitating such actions.

When a person expresses suicidal thoughts or engages in self-harm behaviors (DSH), it serves as a critical distress signal that requires immediate attention from emergency physicians. Suicidal tendencies should be assessed in individuals exhibiting symptoms of depression, unusual behavior changes, substance abuse, psychiatric disorders, or those reporting sexual violence. Additionally, patients with injuries resulting from questionable or inconsistent mechanisms, such as self-inflicted lacerations, gunshot wounds, or motor vehicle accidents involving a single victim, should be thoroughly assessed for suicidal risk. Many experts believe that evaluating self-harm should be a standard component of emergency department (ED) assessments.

A retrospective study by Da Cruz et al. revealed that 40% of individuals who died by suicide had visited the ED at least once in the year prior to their death. This highlights the importance of incorporating comprehensive psychosocial evaluations during emergency care. By discussing the patient's psychosocial situation, healthcare providers can better uncover underlying suicidal ideation or self-harm thoughts, enabling early referral to appropriate support services and providing holistic care to address the individual's needs.

A systematic, multidisciplinary approach is essential for effective assessment. This approach involves staff education, appropriate triage, observation, and restraint protocols for patients at imminent risk, especially when less restrictive options are unavailable. The assessment process should prioritize understanding the physical consequences of the act, the risk of future self-harm behaviors, any psychiatric diagnoses, and acute psychosocial stressors. These factors should be targeted for immediate interventions.

However, risk assessment tools that classify individuals into broad categories (low, medium, or high risk) often fail to predict suicide accurately. The prevalence of suicide is relatively low, and there are a high number of false positives in the "high-risk" groups, with many individuals who later complete suicide classified as "low risk." This underlines the difficulty of accurately predicting suicidal outcomes based solely on risk assessment scales.

Triage and Initial Management

In the case of patients who have attempted self-harm, immediate management must focus on resuscitation, treatment of life-threatening conditions, and preventing further complications. Triage should account for both the physical injuries and the patient's mental state, including current suicidality, agitation, and aggression. A mental health triage scale may be useful in guiding this process. For patients exhibiting violent behavior, active suicidality, psychosis, distress, or the potential to leave the ED prematurely, a triage score of 2 or 3 is appropriate. In such cases, continuous observation by nursing staff or security personnel may be necessary.

Medical Assessment and Safety Measures

To optimize patient safety in the ED, measures should be taken to restrict access to potential self-harm tools, such as sharp objects, medications, ropes, belts, or windows. Hospital gowns can help identify patients attempting to abscond, and increased visibility through security cameras or high-visibility cubicles can further enhance safety. If the patient's assessment is challenging due to medical instability or reluctance to cooperate, anxiolytics may be administered, and physical restraint may be necessary under the duty of care or in extreme situations, following local mental health laws. It's essential that patients, as well as their family and friends, receive emotional support throughout this process, with clear explanations of the rationale behind the decisions and procedures.

Suicide Risk Assessment

The initial suicide risk assessment in the ED should focus on determining the patient's disposition, though a more comprehensive psychiatric evaluation may need to be delayed until the effects of any substances or anxiolytics have worn off. It's crucial to gather collateral information from reliable sources such as family, friends, primary care providers, or past medical records. Establishing a positive, non-judgmental therapeutic relationship with the patient is key. Research indicates that this approach improves outcomes, as patients are more likely to respond positively to care when they feel heard and understood.

Managing patients expressing self-harm ideation requires open discussion, as the meaning of self-harm differs for each individual. The patient's history and current circumstances must be explored to understand the underlying factors contributing to their distress.

Risk Factors

Suicide risk factors are typically divided into static and dynamic categories. Static factors, which include characteristics like gender, employment status, mental health history, and social circumstances, are relatively stable over time. For example, males, the unemployed, socially isolated individuals, and those with a history of mental health or substance use disorders are at higher risk.

Dynamic factors, on the other hand, refer to more immediate conditions such as current emotional distress, substance use, co-occurring mental illness, and external stressors like recent life changes or social dislocation. The interaction between these factors can significantly increase the risk of suicide, highlighting the importance of assessing both types of risk factors. According to Rosenman, no single factor can predict suicide risk, and these factors often interact in unpredictable ways. A person's suicide risk may fluctuate rapidly, particularly in response to acute stressors like intoxication or emotional crises.

Assessment Tools

Several screening tools have been developed to identify individuals at high risk for suicide, such as the PATHOS scale, the Suicidal Intent Scale, and the Sad Persons Scale. However, these tools have limitations. Many rely on outdated risk factors or unrepresentative patient populations, which may lead to misclassification of risk. These scales should not be used as the sole basis for determining the need for psychiatric intervention or hospitalization. Although some validated interview-based tools, like the Suicide Attempt Self-Injury Interview, may offer more accuracy, they are time-consuming and may not always be practical in fast-paced emergency settings.

Risk Stratification and Disposition

After initial medical treatment and suicide risk stratification, patient disposition may involve inpatient psychiatric care, short-term observation, or discharge with appropriate follow-up. High-risk patients who express a desire to self-discharge may require restraint or compulsory admission. For those who are intoxicated, short-term observation allows the effects of substances to wear off before a more comprehensive psychiatric evaluation can be conducted.

Prevention Strategies for Suicide

Suicide prevention strategies have been developed and are actively implemented in countries such as Finland, Norway, Sweden, Australia, and New Zealand. These initiatives focus on various aspects, including psychiatric, social, and medical domains, and generally encompass public awareness campaigns, media guidelines to limit suicide reporting, and school-based programs that educate teachers. Additional preventive measures aim to improve the detection and treatment of mental health issues like depression, alcohol, and drug use, while enhancing access to mental health services and providing support following episodes of deliberate self-harm (DSH).

Furthermore, reducing the availability of methods commonly used in suicides, such as firearms and certain medications, is often a key aspect of legislative efforts. This may involve stricter gun control laws, restricting access to well-known jumping sites, and modifying the packaging of harmful substances. Despite these efforts, research into the effectiveness of suicide prevention strategies has shown mixed results, with only inconsistent reductions in suicide rates post-intervention. Similarly, methods to reduce the recurrence of DSH have generally not yielded significant improvements.

While specific suicide prevention strategies may not be entirely effective, improving the recognition and management of mental health conditions, along with stronger social services and substance abuse support, may provide greater benefit.

Ethical and Governance Considerations

In managing patients presenting with DSH or suicidal ideation, it is essential to balance their autonomy and self-determination with clinical judgment. This includes respecting their wishes, such as refusing recommended treatment or follow-up, while considering their mental state, risk factors, and available support networks (e.g., family, caregivers, financial resources). Ethical concerns also involve evaluating the patient's ability to provide informed consent and ensuring their dignity, particularly when clinicians must initiate immediate care or restrict the patient's autonomy in situations of imminent risk.

In cases of immediate danger, confidentiality may need to be compromised to ensure the patient's safety, as collateral information from healthcare providers, family members, or other involved parties may be necessary. Additionally, local laws governing access to mental health records and electronic databases must be respected when handling sensitive patient information.

The management of patients in emergency departments (EDs) must also take into account healthcare service goals, such as response times and discharge targets. Balancing principles like non-maleficence with utilitarian considerations (e.g., ensuring broader access to care and responsiveness) can sometimes be challenging in the ED setting, where quick decisions are crucial. Adapting services to improve care for suicidal patients is an ongoing process that requires continual evidence-based evaluation.

Emergency departments are required to have written policies for handling suicidal patients. These policies should include evidence-based clinical pathways and protocols for patient observation, searches by medical staff, and the use of physical restraint when necessary.

Conclusion

The assessment of suicide risk is a critical skill for emergency physicians, as many individuals who exhibit suicidal thoughts or behaviors seek care in EDs. Although predicting suicide risk for an individual is complex, emergency departments can provide structured systems for assessing and identifying patients at high risk. Immediate interventions can help prevent suicide or reduce the likelihood of repeated self-harm. During a patient's stay in the ED, connections to long-term support services should be established. A collaborative approach involving psychiatry and social work is often necessary, with many cases resolving through short-term hospitalization, crisis intervention, and intensive follow-up care.

References

1. Salter A, Pielage P. Emergency departments have a role in the prevention of suicide. Emerg Med. 2000;12:198–203.

2. Betz M, Boudreaux D. Managing suicidal patients in the emergency department. Ann Emerg Med. 2016;67(2):276–282.

3. Australian Bureau of Statistics. Causes of Death Australia, 2017. [updated September 2018; cited 2019].

4. National Survey of Mental Health and Wellbeing: Summary of Results; 2007. [Internet homepage] [updated October 2008; cited February 2019].

5. Owens D, Horrocks J, House A. Fatal and non-fatal repetition of self-harm. Br J Psychiatr. 2002;181:193–199.

6. Office of National Statistics, United Kingdom. Statistical Bulletin. Suicide rate in the UK 2006–2010. [Updated January 2012; cited February 2019].

7. New Zealand Ministry of Health, New Zealand. Suicide Facts: Deaths and Intentional Self-Harm. [Updated August 2015; cited February 2019].

Chapter 4
Depression Management and Intervention Strategies

Key Points

1. Prevalence: Clinical depression affects 2% to 5% of individuals at any given time.

2. Assessment: Depressive symptoms can be effectively evaluated through a structured interview and mental state examination.

3. Diagnosis: The diagnosis of depression is based on the severity, pervasiveness, and duration of symptoms.

4. Comorbidities: It is essential to identify common comorbid conditions, such as anxiety and substance use disorders.

5. Treatment Setting: Most cases of depression can be managed effectively within a primary healthcare setting, with specialist care or hospital admission necessary for more severe cases or those with higher risk.

Introduction

Assessing depression is a critical task in the emergency department (ED), as it is often encountered in various patient presentations. Depression must be evaluated in cases of overdose, attempted suicide, or self-harm, typically after the patient has been medically stabilized. It is also increasingly common for patients to seek ED care with depression-related concerns, often encouraged by family, friends, or helplines, without any history of self-harm. Additionally, patients with chronic or disabling medical conditions frequently experience depressive symptoms that contribute to their ED visits. Individuals with personality disorders presenting in the ED are at higher risk for co-occurring depression, particularly when substance abuse is also involved.

The clinical evaluation of depression is based on the concept of 'clinical depression,' which is categorized as 'Major Depression' in the Diagnostic and Statistical Manual of Mental Disorders—5th edition (DSM-5) and as a 'Depressive Episode' in the International Classification of Diseases—10th edition (ICD-10). Diagnosing a depressive episode is crucial as it helps determine the need for treatment, which is likely to be effective and can prevent the persistence of symptoms. Proper diagnosis also allows for differentiation from other medical or psychiatric conditions and distinguishes clinical depression from temporary mood fluctuations, which everyone experiences at times.

The diagnosis of a depressive episode is based on the presence of a prolonged, pervasive change in mood, a marked loss of interest in usual activities, or significant fatigue. Additionally, patients often experience a range of other symptoms, which are detailed in the ICD-10 and DSM-5 diagnostic criteria. These include feelings of worthlessness, guilt, suicidal thoughts, difficulty concentrating, psychomotor changes, changes in sleep or appetite, and weight fluctuations. To be classified as a depressive episode, symptoms must persist for at least two weeks and must significantly impair the patient's daily functioning.

ICD-10 further classifies depressive episodes into three severity categories: mild (4-5 symptoms), moderate (6-7 symptoms), and severe (8 or more symptoms). Even in mild or moderate cases, two of the first three symptoms—depressed mood, loss of interest, and loss of energy—must be present for diagnosis. Severe depression requires all three primary symptoms. The diagnosis is not contingent on the presence of a precipitating event or life stressor, although such events may be relevant in cases of brief depressive reactions or adjustment disorders.

Epidemiology

Depressive episodes, or Major Depression, are widespread, with a 6-month prevalence rate ranging from 2% to 5% across global populations. Despite the high prevalence, many individuals with depression do not receive adequate treatment. The typical onset of a depressive episode occurs in the third decade of life, with a higher incidence among females, with a male-to-female ratio of approximately 1:2. The recurrence rate for depression is notably high, with an 80% chance of recurrence after an initial episode.

Patients with recurrent depression experience, on average, four episodes over their lifetime. Incomplete recovery is common, with 30% of hospitalized patients remaining symptomatic for over a year, and 12% enduring symptoms for more than five years. There is also evidence indicating an increase in both the prevalence of depression and the younger age of onset in recent decades.

Aetiology

The causes of depression are multifactorial, involving genetic and environmental factors. Childhood adversity or neglect and adult life stressors are significant environmental contributors. Genetic factors, particularly inherited tendencies toward excessive worry and anxiety, can also increase susceptibility. Precipitating life events, especially those involving loss, play a role in triggering depressive episodes. However, subsequent episodes are more likely to occur without identifiable triggers, indicating that the first episode may have a neurobiological priming effect.

Research into the neurobiology of depression has evolved from focusing on neurotransmitter depletion to exploring changes in neural populations, particularly in the hippocampus. Antidepressant medications, which target neurotransmitters, suggest that imbalances in brain chemicals may underlie the disorder.

Prevention

Depression is a major public health issue, affecting millions worldwide. The World Health Organization estimates that 322 million people are living with depression, making it the leading cause of disability globally. Public health initiatives have raised awareness of depression, aiming to reduce stigma and improve diagnosis and treatment. Emergency department staff play a critical role in identifying patients with depression and ensuring appropriate referrals for treatment.

Clinical Features

The clinical presentation of Major Depression is defined by specific symptoms that affect mood, cognition, and physical functioning. The severity of the episode depends on the number, intensity, and duration of these symptoms. When assessing a patient in the ED, it is essential to understand the context of their symptoms, including any underlying medical conditions, personal crises, or recent life events.

The assessment typically begins by understanding the presenting issue—such as a suicide attempt, self-harm, relationship crisis, or chronic medical condition exacerbation. The patient's living situation, social relationships, occupation, and activities also provide valuable context for understanding the severity and implications of their depressive symptoms.

Once the broader context is established, the clinician should explore the patient's depressive symptoms in detail, grouping them into categories: mood state (depressed mood, loss of interest, loss of energy), cognitive symptoms (self-esteem issues, guilt, suicidal thoughts), physical manifestations (concentration problems, psychomotor changes), and physiological changes (sleep disturbances, appetite changes). This helps in forming a complete picture of the patient's experience and severity of the disorder.

Symptoms must be present "most of the day" and "nearly every day" for at least two weeks to meet the diagnostic criteria. Functionality is another key indicator of severity—patients may experience increasing difficulty in managing daily tasks, ranging from work or childcare to personal hygiene and nutrition. This functional impairment is a crucial factor in determining the impact of depression on the patient's life.

The onset of depression can be gradual or sudden, making it challenging to determine the exact beginning of the episode. Patients often confuse long-standing feelings of low self-esteem with more recent depressive episodes. Therefore, clinicians should inquire about the patient's symptoms over the past two to three weeks, noting any recent changes in their emotional or functional state. This approach helps in identifying the onset and progression of the depressive episode, enabling a more accurate diagnosis and appropriate treatment plan.

Signs and Features of Depression: Detailed Analysis

Key Signs:

The primary indicators of depression include:

Psychomotor agitation or retardation

The patient's affective state

Thought content

Level of insight

Psychomotor Agitation:
Patients experiencing psychomotor agitation exhibit restless or repetitive behaviors such as hand-wringing or sighing. Milder cases involve fidgety actions, escalating to an inability to remain still, culminating in continuous pacing. These individuals may appear visibly anxious and ask repetitive questions in search of reassurance, which is

seldom achieved. In severe agitation, speech becomes repetitive and unproductive.

Psychomotor Retardation:
Conversely, psychomotor-retarded individuals demonstrate significant immobility, often sitting or lying in one position for extended periods. Facial expressions may be blank, appearing sad or anxious, with limited reactivity during interactions. Verbal communication is minimal and lacks depth or spontaneity. Severe cases may involve muteness and pronounced delays in responding to questions.

Affective State:
Depressed patients typically present with sadness but may also exhibit anxiety or hostility. As the condition worsens, emotional expression diminishes, and patients become unresponsive to positive social cues, such as smiling.

Thought Content:
Patients often discuss themes of despair, guilt, failure, or preoccupation with death. These thought patterns align closely with depressive episodes.

Insight:
The degree of insight, or the patient's awareness of their condition, often correlates with the severity of depression.

Variants of Depression

Melancholic Depression:
Severe depressive episodes with prominent physiological disturbances and psychomotor symptoms are classified as melancholic depression. Diagnostic criteria such as those in the DSM-5 (Major Depression with Melancholic Features) and ICD-10 (Depressive Episode with Somatic

Syndrome) emphasize at least four symptoms, including:

1. Loss of pleasure in most activities

2. Lack of emotional response to typically pleasurable events

3. Early morning awakening

4. Worsening depression in the morning

5. Marked psychomotor agitation or retardation

6. Significant appetite loss or weight loss (>5% of body weight)

7. Decreased libido

Clinical Significance:
Melancholic depression often necessitates intensive biological treatment, as it involves

more severe and specific forms of typical depressive symptoms.

Psychotic Depression:
This form involves severe depressive episodes with psychotic features, such as delusions or hallucinations, and typically meets criteria for somatic syndrome.

Mild and Moderate Depressive Episodes

Recognizing milder forms of depression may be more challenging, particularly in patients with long-standing low self-esteem or a predisposition to worry or irritability. While these temperamental factors may influence presentation, the defining feature of a depressive episode is a persistent mood change lasting at least two weeks.

Common Symptoms:

Depressed mood

Loss of interest

Low energy

Sleep disturbances

Impaired concentration

Functional impairment is a reliable indicator. Questions assessing daily activities, such as household tasks, work performance, and leisure participation, can reveal the extent of disruption caused by depressive symptoms.

Special Populations

Elderly:
Depression in older adults resembles that in younger populations but may be masked by coexisting medical conditions. Persistent mood changes or loss of interest should

prompt evaluation. Symptoms like cognitive changes, termed "pseudodementia," may also occur, characterized by heightened awareness of memory difficulties and anxiety.

Brief Depressive Reactions:
This category describes depressive symptoms arising from stressful life events, such as interpersonal conflicts, without meeting criteria for a depressive episode. Symptoms are transient and may improve with distraction or supportive therapy.

Grief:
Grief shares overlapping symptoms with depression, such as mood disturbance and sleep issues. However, if symptoms persist beyond six months or significantly impair function, a depressive episode should be considered.

Differential Diagnosis

Bipolar Depression:
A history of manic or hypomanic episodes differentiates bipolar depression from unipolar depression. This distinction is crucial, as treatment approaches differ significantly, with antidepressants used cautiously in bipolar patients to avoid inducing mania.

Organic Mood Disorders:
Depressive syndromes secondary to medical conditions (e.g., hypothyroidism, hyperparathyroidism, pancreatic cancer, or neurological diseases like Huntington's or HIV/AIDS) require thorough evaluation. In some cases, depression may be the first manifestation of an underlying illness.

Diagnostic Considerations

The evaluation of depressive episodes must account for comorbidities, functional impairment, and psychosocial context. By focusing on objective signs such as psychomotor changes, affective reactivity, and persistent mood alterations, clinicians can accurately distinguish depression from other conditions, ensuring appropriate treatment and management.

Chronic Dysthymia

Dysthymia is a persistent, low-grade depressive disorder characterized by a long-standing sense of dissatisfaction with life, lack of enjoyment, and a generally gloomy or pessimistic outlook. Patients often exhibit personality traits intertwined with depressive tendencies, such as chronic self-criticism, low self-esteem, and diminished motivation. Unlike major depressive episodes, dysthymia does not meet the full diagnostic criteria for severe depressive disorders. The condition typically begins in early adulthood and can persist for several years. Epidemiological studies estimate its prevalence to be approximately 3% of the general population.

An exacerbation of dysthymia symptoms may lead to the development of a major depressive episode, a phenomenon referred to as "double depression." Patients with dysthymia might present to emergency departments (EDs) with suicidal thoughts or behaviors. Given its chronic nature and significant impact on mental health, early referral to psychiatric or mental health services is crucial for management. Treatment is often complex and may require a multidisciplinary approach.

Anxiety Disorders

Anxiety disorders encompass various conditions, including panic disorder (recurrent panic attacks), generalized anxiety disorder (GAD) (persistent worrying with somatic symptoms such as muscle tension), obsessive-compulsive disorder

(OCD), and specific phobias (e.g., agoraphobia or social phobia). In many cases, anxiety symptoms overlap with depressive symptoms, making differentiation between primary anxiety disorders and depressive disorders challenging, especially in emergency settings.

Patients with primary anxiety disorders often report a long history of symptoms, sometimes spanning months or years, and may concurrently develop depressive syndromes. The coexistence of anxiety and depression is common, complicating diagnosis and treatment. When assessing such patients in EDs, the presence of persistent depressed mood and suicidal ideation often necessitates inpatient treatment. Conversely, patients without these severe symptoms may be safely referred to their primary care physician or outpatient mental health services for further evaluation.

Personality Disorders

Personality disorders involve deeply ingrained, enduring patterns of behavior and interpersonal interactions that deviate significantly from cultural norms and are associated with distress or conflict. These patterns are typically evident from adolescence or early adulthood.

Common Types in Emergency Settings:

1. Antisocial Personality Disorder (ASPD): Individuals with ASPD frequently exhibit a disregard for societal norms, resulting in unstable employment, broken relationships, and sometimes violent or criminal behavior. They may present to EDs due to crises, brief depressive reactions, or suicidal ideation. Assessment should determine whether a superimposed depressive episode is present and assess its severity.

Inpatient treatment can be challenging due to noncompliance with structured settings, but crisis counseling or outpatient therapy may provide more feasible interventions.

2. Borderline Personality Disorder (BPD):
BPD is marked by erratic interpersonal relationships, impulsivity, and emotional instability. Patients often experience chronic feelings of emptiness, self-harm behaviors, and intense reactions to perceived rejection or abandonment. While these features may mimic depression, they are often intrinsic to the personality disorder rather than indicative of a distinct depressive episode. Approximately 50% of individuals with BPD may meet criteria for a depressive episode at any given time. Crisis intervention in EDs should focus on connecting patients to outpatient services to ensure continuity of care.

Comprehensive Assessment

Evaluating patients presenting with depressive symptoms involves:

Exploring social context: living arrangements, relationships, employment, and support systems.

Investigating recent stressors or triggers.

Conducting a systematic assessment of depressive symptoms, including severity and persistence.

Reviewing psychiatric history, including prior depressive or manic episodes, and response to past treatments.

Performing a mental state examination to evaluate mood, psychomotor activity, and thought content (e.g., guilt, failure, or death themes).

Conducting a risk assessment for suicide or self-harm, including protective factors and aggravating circumstances.

Additionally, clinicians should consider medical conditions or substance use contributing to depressive symptoms. Relevant laboratory tests (e.g., thyroid function and hemoglobin levels) may aid in excluding medical causes.

Treatment Approaches

Pharmacotherapy

Antidepressant medications are a cornerstone of treatment. Selective serotonin reuptake inhibitors (SSRIs), such as fluoxetine and sertraline, are commonly first-line options due to their favorable side-effect profiles. However, long-term side effects, such as sexual dysfunction, may necessitate alternative treatments. Other options include:

Serotonin-noradrenaline reuptake inhibitors (SNRIs): Effective but associated with additional side effects like excessive sweating and withdrawal symptoms upon discontinuation.

Mirtazapine: Useful for patients with insomnia or agitation but may lead to weight gain.

Psychotherapy

Evidence-based psychotherapeutic interventions, such as cognitive-behavioral therapy (CBT) and interpersonal therapy (IPT), are often combined with medication for optimal outcomes.

Conclusion

Effective management of depressive and anxiety disorders, as well as personality disorders, requires a thorough assessment, accurate diagnosis, and a tailored treatment plan. Early intervention and appropriate referrals play a pivotal role in improving patient outcomes, especially for those presenting in crisis.

References

1. World Health Organization. ICD-10: Classification of Mental and Behavioral Disorders. Geneva: World Health Organization; 1993.

2. American Psychiatric Association. Diagnostic and Statistical Manual of Mental Disorders. 5th ed. Arlington, VA: American Psychiatric Association; 2013.

3. GBD 2016 Disease and Injury Incidence and Prevalence Collaborators. Global, regional, and national data on the incidence, prevalence, and disability for 328 diseases and injuries across 195 countries from 1990 to 2016: A systematic analysis for the Global Burden of Disease Study 2016. The Lancet. 2017;390(10100):1211–1259.

4. Markkula N, Suvisaari J. Prevalence, risk factors, and prognosis associated with depressive disorders. Duodecim. 2017;133(3):275–282.

5. Katz M, Secunda S, Hirschfeld R. Overview of the NIMH clinical research program on the psychobiology of depression. Archives of General Psychiatry. 1979;36:765–771.

6. Cross-National Collaborative Group. Trends in the prevalence of major depression: A comparative analysis across

nations. Journal of the American Medical Association. 1992;268:3098–3105.

7. Tennant C. A review of life events, stress, and their role in depression. Australian and New Zealand Journal of Psychiatry. 2002;36:173–182.

8. Frank E, Anderson B, Reynolds C. Life events and endogenous subtypes based on research diagnostic criteria. Archives of General Psychiatry. 1994;51:519–524.

9. Kendler K, Thornton L, Gardner C. An evaluation of the 'kindling' hypothesis in the context of major depression etiology among women. American Journal of Psychiatry. 2000;157:1243–1251.

10. Schildkraut J. Review of the catecholamine hypothesis in affective disorders. American Journal of Psychiatry. 1965;122:509–522.

11. Jacobs B, van Praag H, Gage F. Insights into adult brain neurogenesis and its implications in psychiatric disorders: A novel theory of depression. Molecular Psychiatry. 2000;5:262–269.

12. World Health Organization. Depression and Other Common Mental Disorders: Global Health Estimates. Geneva: World Health Organization; 2017.

13. Parker G, Hadzi-Pavlovic D. Melancholia: A Disorder of Movement and Mood. Cambridge: Cambridge University Press; 1996.

14. Yoon S, Dang V, Mertz J, Rottenberg J. The relationship between attitudes towards emotions and depression: A conceptual and meta-analytic review. Journal of Affective Disorders. 2018;232:329–340.

15. Tunvirachaisakul C, Gould RL, Coulson MC, et al. A systematic review and

meta-analysis of predictors influencing depression treatment outcomes in later life. Journal of Affective Disorders. 2018;227:164–182.

16. Lindemann E. Acute grief: Symptomatology and management. American Journal of Psychiatry. 1944;101:141.

17. Gold M, Pottash A, Extein I. Association between hypothyroidism and depressive disorders. Journal of the American Medical Association. 1981;245:1919–1922.

18. Watson L. Clinical characteristics of hyperparathyroidism. Proceedings of the Royal Society of Medicine. 1968;61:1123.

19. Joffe R, Rubinow D, Denicoff K. Depression as a symptom in pancreatic carcinoma. General Hospital Psychiatry. 1986;8:241–245.

20. Folstein S, Abbott M, Chase G. Affective disorders in Huntington's disease: Findings from case series and familial studies. Psychological Medicine. 1983;13:537–542.

21. Atkinson J, Grant I, Kennedy C. Prevalence of psychiatric conditions in HIV-positive men. Archives of General Psychiatry. 1988;45:859–864.

22. Hales R, Yudofsky S. The American Psychiatric Publishing Textbook of Clinical Psychiatry. 4th ed. Washington, DC: American Psychiatric Publishing; 2003:462–463.

23. Cornelius J, Salloumi, Ehler J. Fluoxetine's efficacy in reducing depression and alcohol consumption among patients with comorbid conditions. Archives of General Psychiatry. 1997;54:700–705.

24. Akiskal H, Cassano G, editors. Dysthymia and the Spectrum of Chronic

Depressions. New York: Guilford Press; 1997.

25. Waintraub L, Guelfi J. Dysthymia: Historical, epidemiological, and clinical data supporting its nosological validity. European Psychiatry. 1998;13:173–180.

26. Haykal R, Akiskal H. The clinical features, temperament, and management strategies in the long-term outcomes of dysthymia. Journal of Clinical Psychiatry. 1999;60:508–518.

27. Gunderson J. Borderline Personality Disorder: A Clinical Guide. Washington, DC: American Psychiatric Publishing; 2001.

28. Seligman M. Learned Optimism. New York: Random House; 1991.

29. Weissman M, Markowitz J, Klerman G. Comprehensive Guide to Interpersonal

Psychotherapy. New York: Basic Books; 2000.

30. Harris R. Acceptance and commitment therapy: An overview. Psychotherapy in Australia. 2006;12.

31. Chiesa A, Serretti A. A systematic review and meta-analysis of mindfulness-based cognitive therapy in psychiatric disorders. Psychiatry Research. 2011;187:441–453.

32. Mali G, Bassett D, Boyce P, et al. Mood disorders clinical guidelines by the Royal Australian and New Zealand College of Psychiatrists. Australian and New Zealand Journal of Psychiatry. 2015;49:1–185.

33. Paykel E, Scott J, Gelder M, et al. Treatment approaches for mood disorders. In: Gelder M, Lopez-Ibor J, Andreasen N, editors. New Oxford Textbook of Psychiatry.

Oxford: Oxford University Press; 2007:24–726.

34. Eaton W, Anthony J, Gallo G. A follow-up study on DSM-IV major depression in the Baltimore Epidemiologic Catchment Area. Archives of General Psychiatry. 1997;54:993–999.

35. Wijkstra J, Lijmer J, Burger H, et al. Efficacy of pharmacological treatments for psychotic depression: A systematic review. Cochrane Database of Systematic Reviews. 2015;7:CD004044.

36. Dobson K. Cognitive therapy for depression: A meta-analytic review of its efficacy. Journal of Consulting and Clinical Psychology. 1988;57:414–419.

37. Lampe L, Coulston C, Berk L. Psychological management strategies for unipolar depression. Acta Psychiatrica

Scandinavica Supplement. 2013;(443):24–37.

38. Driessen E, Cuijpers P, Hollon SD, Dekker JJ. Moderating effects of pretreatment severity on psychological treatments for adult depression: A meta-analysis. Journal of Consulting and Clinical Psychology. 2010;78:668.

Chapter 5
Psychosis

Key Points

1. Emergency Department as a Crucial Assessment Site
With the shift towards community mental health care, emergency departments play a pivotal role in evaluating patients presenting with psychosis.

2. Differentiating Psychosis from Organic Causes
Clinicians in emergency settings must thoroughly assess for delirium and organic causes of psychotic symptoms, including substance intoxication, to ensure accurate diagnosis and management.

3. Risks Associated with Acute Psychosis

Acute psychosis poses significant risks, including self-harm, suicide, aggression, accidents, and homelessness. Effective disposition decisions—such as referrals to community care or hospitalization—require comprehensive assessments of treatment history, support systems, risk factors, and the patient's mental state and preferences.

4. Collaborative Treatment Planning
Wherever feasible, treatment planning should actively involve patients experiencing psychosis and their caregivers to ensure shared decision-making and enhanced care outcomes.

Introduction

Psychotic disorders are a frequent cause of presentations to emergency departments (EDs), accounting for a significant portion of the workload due to the severity of the patients' mental health conditions. In

Australia, approximately 64,000 individuals aged 18 to 64 with psychotic disorders interact with public specialized mental health services annually. This prevalence translates to 5 cases per 1,000 individuals or 0.5% of the population. Patients experiencing psychotic episodes are often severely mentally ill and typically present to the ED following major crises at home or in the community, often unwillingly.

Managing psychotic patients in the ED presents unique challenges for staff. These tasks include containment and stabilization of agitated or frightened patients, managing behavioral disturbances to mitigate risks to the patient, staff, or others, and performing comprehensive medical assessments to rule out underlying physical conditions. Treatment planning must involve consideration of patient preferences, the potential need for voluntary or involuntary admission, or referrals to community-based services. Engaging family members and caregivers in both assessment and treatment decisions is also critical to achieving optimal outcomes.

Classification

Historically, psychotic disorders were classified into "functional" (non-organic) and "organic" psychoses. Advances in psychiatric classification systems, such as the ICD-10 Classification of Mental and Behavioral Disorders, have broadened this framework, encompassing over 16 diagnostic categories with numerous subtypes for describing psychotic symptoms. However, in the ED, practical classifications focus on immediate priorities:

1. Ruling out medical causes for psychosis.

2. Evaluating the role of substance use (alcohol or drugs).

3. Formulating a provisional psychiatric diagnosis to guide initial treatment.

4. Assessing if the psychosis stems primarily from psychological stress.

These classifications help streamline emergency interventions and set the foundation for further diagnostic refinement.

Epidemiology and Prognosis

Among the primary non-organic psychotic conditions encountered are schizophrenia and bipolar I disorder:

Schizophrenia affects about 1% of the adult population globally, with equal prevalence among men and women. Onset generally occurs before age 30, though it is slightly later in women. The disease course is variable:

Approximately 20% of patients experience significant recovery.

Another 20% have recurrent episodes with full interepisode recovery.

About 40% suffer recurrent episodes with incomplete remission.

The remaining 20% experience severe, chronic symptoms.

Schizophrenia is associated with a high suicide risk, with a 20-year suicide rate of 14–22%.

Bipolar I Disorder has a prevalence of 1%, with an equal gender distribution. Onset typically occurs in late adolescence, with 95% of cases beginning before age 26. Recurrence is common, with an 80% likelihood of another manic episode within five years. Although most patients recover well between episodes, the suicide rate remains significant at 13% over 22 years.

Aetiology and Prevention

The causes of schizophrenia and bipolar disorder remain poorly understood, though genetic and environmental factors play significant roles. For example:

Having one parent with schizophrenia or bipolar disorder increases an individual's risk to about 10%.

Despite advances in understanding, no strategies for primary prevention have been established. However, secondary prevention through early diagnosis and prompt intervention has shown promise. Key strategies include:

Educating patients and families on early warning signs of relapse.

Promoting adherence to maintenance and prophylactic treatments.

Encouraging continuous engagement with mental health services.

Emergency department personnel can play a vital role by emphasizing treatment continuity and facilitating access to specialist care.

Clinical Features

Psychotic symptoms due to general medical conditions should always be ruled out in ED settings. Common causes include:

1. Delirium: Often presenting with visual illusions and persecutory delusions, delirium is characterized by disorientation and fluctuating consciousness. Delirium is

common in older patients or those with sudden onset psychotic symptoms.

2. Dementia: Psychotic symptoms in dementia include hallucinations and persecutory delusions, commonly observed in conditions like Alzheimer's disease.

3. Psychosis with clear consciousness: Rarely, medical conditions such as epilepsy, thyroid dysfunction, or vitamin deficiencies may trigger psychosis without accompanying cognitive impairments.

Psychosis related to prescribed medications also warrants attention. For example:

Steroid psychosis is often dose-dependent and manifests with manic-like symptoms.

Dopamine agonists (e.g., levodopa) used in Parkinson's disease can lead to visual and auditory hallucinations or delusions.

Psychotic Symptoms and Related Syndromes

Manic Syndrome in Bipolar Disorder

Manic syndrome is a recognized presentation of bipolar disorder, alongside depressive episodes and mixed affective states. The classic manic presentation is strikingly characteristic, with individuals typically exhibiting an elevated or irritable mood, rapid and continuous speech (difficult to interrupt), heightened distractibility, and uninhibited or overly familiar behavior. If delusions accompany these symptoms, they often involve grandiosity, such as believing in a significant mission, or paranoia, such as perceiving a conspiracy thwarting their purpose.

Collateral information frequently reveals a sudden onset of symptoms within a few days, including hyperactivity, disorganization, and a reduced need for sleep.

Mixed Affective Psychosis

In mixed affective states, patients display manic-like arousal and irritability combined with depressive themes evident in their speech. This contrasts with purely depressive psychosis, which is discussed separately.

Delirium Versus Mania

Delirium can sometimes mimic mania due to affective instability, irritability, disinhibition, and distractibility. This is particularly seen in older patients without a prior bipolar history. The distinction lies in cognitive dysfunction, such as disorientation, fluctuating alertness, and memory deficits, often coupled with evidence of underlying medical illness.

Mania Versus Acute Schizophrenia

Differentiating acute mania from acute schizophrenia in emergencies can be challenging, especially in first-episode cases. However, immediate and short-term management strategies are generally similar.

Psychotic Depression

Psychotic depression is characterized by severe depressive episodes accompanied by delusions or hallucinations tied to feelings of guilt, worthlessness, or suicidal ideation. This irrationality places patients at high risk for suicide, necessitating close supervision.

Clinical assessment typically reveals a withdrawn, low-energy individual who may also appear agitated or irritable. Differential diagnoses and treatment protocols for depressive syndromes are explored in detail elsewhere.

Substance-Induced Psychosis

Psychotic episodes can result from substance use in several contexts: acute intoxication, withdrawal reactions, prolonged drug abuse leading to chronic psychosis, and exacerbation of pre-existing psychotic disorders. Substances associated with these phenomena include amphetamines, cocaine, phencyclidine, LSD, ketamine, cannabis, alcohol, and benzodiazepines.

1. Acute Intoxication Psychosis: Manifests as hallucinations (auditory and visual), delusions (grandiose or paranoid), agitation, anxiety, and autonomic symptoms such as dilated pupils. Specific substances like phencyclidine can trigger extreme aggression or disinhibition. Treatment

involves ensuring safety and managing acute symptoms until the substance clears.

2. Withdrawal-Related Psychosis: Particularly seen with alcohol and benzodiazepines, withdrawal can induce visual hallucinations and psychosis that improve with appropriate withdrawal management using benzodiazepines.

3. Chronic Substance-Induced Psychosis: Prolonged use of amphetamines and similar drugs can result in enduring psychosis, persisting for weeks or months after cessation. Patients may experience paranoid delusions (e.g., being watched) or hallucinations (e.g., auditory commentary or tactile sensations). Cannabis use often exacerbates psychosis in predisposed individuals.

Reactive Psychotic-Like States

Severe personality disorders, PTSD, or dissociative disorders can precipitate reactive quasi-psychotic episodes, often triggered by acute stress or trauma. These patients may experience vivid traumatic recall, internal monologues perceived as auditory hallucinations, or intense fears resembling paranoia. Emergency management focuses on containment and sedation using benzodiazepines or antipsychotics.

Assessment of Psychotic Patients

In an emergency setting, assessing psychosis involves addressing several key questions:

Is the altered state due to a medical condition?

Are drugs or alcohol contributing factors?

Can a primary psychiatric diagnosis be established?

Is hospitalization required, and should it be involuntary?

Effective assessment requires a holistic approach, incorporating:

Patient history from family or mental health services.

Clinical observation of mental state, speech patterns, and behavior.

Risk evaluation for self-harm or harm to others.

Initial Stabilization and Management

Engaging the psychotic patient calmly and respectfully is critical. Observational assessment can provide valuable insights even when formal evaluations are impractical. Agitation or aggression necessitates safety measures, including security presence, a safe environment, and potential sedation.

Mental State Examination

Observation forms the backbone of the examination, with attention to:

Appearance and self-care.

Speech patterns and thought coherence.

Emotional states (e.g., hostility, euphoria).

Cognitive function, including orientation and memory.

Risk Assessment

Directly addressing suicidal or homicidal ideation is essential, but broader context—social circumstances, family dynamics, and the patient's insight—shapes the overall risk evaluation. Decisions about hospitalization and potential involuntary detention are based on these comprehensive assessments.

Comprehensive Medical and Psychiatric Evaluation in Emergency Settings: A Case-Based Approach

Medical Evaluation and Investigation

The primary objectives of a thorough medical evaluation are threefold: to rule out delirium or dementia, identify organic causes of psychosis, and detect any coexisting medical conditions. However, relying solely on the concept of "medical clearance" before psychiatric evaluation can compromise a holistic assessment. A better approach integrates the following:

1. History and Mental State: Document the history of the presenting illness and assess the mental state.

2. Medication and Substance Use: Review prescribed medications, alcohol, and other substances.

3. Physical Examination: Conduct a detailed examination, emphasizing signs of trauma, poisoning, or intoxication, alongside monitoring vital signs.

Collaborative discussions between emergency physicians and psychiatrists in cases of diagnostic uncertainty are particularly beneficial.

Medical causes for altered mental states often emerge from clinical findings such as history, mental state abnormalities, abnormal vital signs, and physical examination. In older patients or first psychotic episodes, medical etiologies warrant closer scrutiny.

Diagnostic Investigations

Investigations should be guided by clinical findings, including neurological signs or indicators of infection. Due to challenges in obtaining comprehensive medical histories, basic screening tests are commonly performed. These typically include:

Urea and electrolytes

Full blood count

Liver function tests

Blood sugar levels

Thyroid function tests

Vitamin B12 and folate levels

Advancements in computed tomography (CT) availability have made neuroimaging accessible for diagnosing conditions like stroke, tumors, hemorrhages, or infections of the central nervous system (CNS). While neuroimaging is less frequently required in younger patients, it remains valuable for first-episode psychosis when neurological disorders are suspected.

Chronic Psychotic Illness and Comorbidities

Chronic psychotic disorders are frequently accompanied by poor physical health due to factors such as lifestyle choices, medication side effects, and limited access to primary care. Common conditions include obesity, diabetes, hypertension, and substance use disorders. Recognizing and addressing these can significantly improve patient outcomes and mental health stability.

Emergency Department Management

Psychiatric Diagnoses in the ED

Once medical causes are excluded, psychiatric conditions encountered in the emergency department (ED) typically fall into categories such as:

Drug-induced psychosis

Acute schizophrenia

Mania

Chronic schizophrenia

Psychosis-like reactive states

Depressive psychosis

Extended ED stays for psychotic patients often result from assessment delays or lack of available psychiatric beds. To address this, some facilities have introduced specialized psychiatric observation units where patients can receive care and observation for up to 48 hours.

Behavioral and Pharmacological Interventions

Managing behavioral disturbances requires balancing patient safety with minimal restrictions. Strategies include:

Environment: Place patients in quiet, easily monitored areas with trained mental health staff.

Engagement: Encourage reality-based conversations to provide reassurance and orientation.

Family Support: Involve family members when appropriate for comfort and reassurance.

Pharmacological Management:
The choice of medication depends on the underlying diagnosis:

1. Drug-Induced Psychosis: Benzodiazepines like diazepam or midazolam are preferred for sedation, minimizing medical complications.

2. Acute Schizophrenia or Mania: Sedative antipsychotics (e.g., olanzapine) or benzodiazepines (e.g., lorazepam) are used in divided doses to maintain consistent sedation.

3. Psychotic Depression: Low doses of sedative antipsychotics or benzodiazepines are recommended to manage distress and agitation.

4. Reactive Psychosis: Benzodiazepines or antipsychotics can help reduce arousal in patients with personality disorders or trauma history.

Admission and Community Referral

Admission Criteria

Admission decisions depend on the severity of symptoms, risk factors, home support, and access to community mental health services:

Acute Schizophrenia: Admission is often necessary, especially for first episodes due to high risks of disorganization, non-compliance, and self-harm.

Mania: Most patients require admission for stabilization over several weeks.

Psychotic Depression: Admission is critical due to a high risk of suicide.

Chronic Schizophrenia: Community management is preferred when symptoms are mild and adequate support systems are in place.

Involuntary Treatment

When patients refuse admission despite evident risks, involuntary treatment under mental health legislation may be required. Decisions must weigh the risks of untreated conditions against the availability of community resources and family support. Mental health specialists should oversee these decisions whenever possible.

Community-Based Care

The increasing availability of mobile crisis teams has made outpatient care feasible for many patients. Early discharge with robust community follow-up, including mental health team involvement, is preferred for stable patients.

Conclusion

Effective management of psychiatric emergencies requires an integrative approach that prioritizes both physical and mental health. Comprehensive assessments, judicious use of pharmacological interventions, and careful admission decisions contribute to improved outcomes for individuals experiencing psychosis or related conditions.

References

1. Morgan VA, Waterreus A, Jablensky A, et al. People Living with Psychotic Illness 2010. Canberra: Australian Government Department of Health and Ageing; 2012.

2. Kalucy R, Thomas L, King D. Examining shifting patterns in demand for mental health services in public hospital emergency departments. Aust NZ J Psychiatry. 2005;39:74–80.

3. World Health Organization. The ICD-10 Classification of Mental and Behavioural Disorders. Geneva: WHO; 1993.

4. Jablensky A, Gelder MG, Lopez-Ibor JJ, Andreasen NC. Epidemiological insights into schizophrenia. In: Gelder MG, Lopez-Ibor JJ, Andreasen NC, editors. New Oxford Textbook of Psychiatry. London: New Oxford Press; 2000.

5. Jablensky A, Gelder MG, Lopez-Ibor JJ, Andreasen NC. Predicting the progression and outcomes of schizophrenia. In: Gelder MG, Lopez-Ibor JJ, Andreasen NC, editors. New Oxford Textbook of Psychiatry. London: New Oxford Press; 2000.

6. Joyce PR, Gelder MG, Lopez-Ibor JJ, Andreasen NC. Prevalence and distribution of mood disorders. In: Gelder MG, Lopez-Ibor JJ, Andreasen NC, editors. New Oxford Textbook of Psychiatry. London: New Oxford Press; 2000.

7. Angst J, Gelder MG, Lopez-Ibor JJ, Andreasen NC. Mood disorders: course and prognosis. In: Gelder MG, Lopez-Ibor JJ, Andreasen NC, editors. New Oxford Textbook of Psychiatry. London: New Oxford Press; 2000.

8. McGorry PD. Secondary prevention and recovery frameworks in psychiatric

disorders. Aust NZ J Psychiatry. 1992;26:3–17.

9. Douglas S, Ballard C, Hassett A, et al. Psychotic symptoms in dementia. In: Hassett A, Ames D, Chiu E, editors. Psychosis in the Elderly. London: Taylor & Francis; 2005.

10. Brudekjoler SR, Mortensen PB, Parnas J. A national epidemiological study on epilepsy and non-organic psychosis. Br J Psychiatry. 1998;172:235–238.

11. Maguire M, Singh J, Marson A. Epilepsy-associated psychosis: clinical approaches. Pract Neurol. 2018;18(2):106–114.

12. Hales RH, Yudofsky SC. Textbook of Clinical Psychiatry. 4th ed. Washington, DC: American Psychiatric Publishing; 2003:462–463.

13. Boston Collaborative Drug Surveillance Program. Acute adverse effects of prednisolone: dosage correlations. Clin Pharmacol Ther. 1972;13:694–698.

14. Taylor J, Anderson WS, Brandt J, et al. Neuropsychiatric issues in Parkinson's treatment: emphasizing interdisciplinary care. Am J Geriatr Psychiatry. 2016;24(12):1171–1180.

15. Mellor CS. Defining first-rank symptoms of schizophrenia. Br J Psychiatry. 1970;117:15–23.

16. Bramness JG, Rognli EB. Amphetamine-induced psychosis: insights and developments. Curr Opin Psychiatry. 2016;29(4):236–241.

17. Holtzman CW, Trotman HD, Goulding SM, et al. Stress and neurodevelopmental factors in psychosis onset. Neuroscience. 2013;249:172–191.

18. Abraham HD, Aldridge AM, Gogia P. Psychopharmacology of hallucinogens: a review. Neuropsychopharmacology. 1996;14:285–298.

19. Hall W. Cannabis and its association with psychosis. Drug Alcohol Rev. 1998;17:433–434.

20. Chopra HD, Beatson JA. Psychotic manifestations in borderline personality disorder. Am J Psychiatry. 1986;143:1605–1607.

21. Butler RW, Mueser KT, Sprock J. Positive psychotic symptoms linked to PTSD. Biol Psychiatry. 1996;39:839–844.

22. Janiak BD, Atteberry S. Psychiatric patient evaluation for medical clearance in emergency settings. J Emerg Med. 2012;43(5):866–870.

23. Thienhaus OH, Hillard JP. Physical assessment and laboratory testing. In: Hillard JP, editor. Manual of Clinical Emergency Psychiatry. Washington, DC: American Psychiatric Press; 1990.

24. Rock DJ, Wynn Owen P. Investigating criteria for cranial CT in males diagnosed with schizophrenia. Acta Neuropsychiatr. 2003;15:284–289.

25. Albon E, Tsourapas A, Frew E, et al. Structural neuroimaging in psychosis: systematic review and economic analysis. Health Technol Assess. 2008;12(18):3–4, 9–163.

26. Phelan M, Stradius L, Morrison S. Physical health challenges in individuals with severe mental illnesses. Br Med J. 2001;322:443–444.

27. Allen MM. Crisis intervention tools in psychiatric emergency services. Psychiatr Clin N Am. 1999;22:713–733.

28. Frank R, Fawcett L, Emmerson B. The evolution of Australia's first psychiatric emergency center. Aust Psychiatry. 2005;13:266–272.

29. Bennett C, Fumall J, Fossey E, et al. Meeting the needs of individuals with schizophrenia and related disorders. In: Meadow G, Singh B, editors. Mental Health in Australia: Collaborative Community Practice. Melbourne: Oxford University Press; 2001:283–312.

30. Breslow RE. The structure and operational dynamics of psychiatric emergency services. In: Allen M, editor. Emergency Psychiatry. Washington, DC: American Psychiatric Press; 2002.

Chapter 6
Pharmacological Approaches to Managing Patient Agitation

Key Points

1. First-Line Medications: Benzodiazepines and antipsychotics are commonly used in combination as the primary drugs for sedation of an agitated patient.

2. Pre-Sedation Assessment: It is essential to gather as much relevant information as possible before administering sedation.

3. Risk Considerations: The potential risks associated with sedative drugs, especially at higher doses, must be carefully evaluated.

4. Dose Adjustments: Adjustments in medication dosage are crucial for older

adults and patients with medical comorbidities to avoid complications.

Introduction

When patients present in an agitated or aroused state to the emergency department (ED), those who arrive voluntarily generally respond best to verbal reassurance and a prompt mental health assessment. Minimizing their waiting time and swiftly formulating an action plan can significantly alleviate anxiety and agitation. For patients who are brought in against their will, the priority is to gain control of the situation to ensure the safety of the patient, staff, and public, while preparing for further evaluation.

Before proceeding with sedation, it is preferable to gather some basic patient information. The patient should be approached calmly in a safe and monitored area of the ED, with security on standby if necessary. Engaging the patient by asking them to explain their understanding of the situation, even if their account seems incoherent, can provide reassurance and foster rapport. This approach also offers an opportunity to observe the patient's mental state. If possible, vital signs should be recorded, and a brief physical exam should be performed, focusing on potential injuries, signs of intoxication, or overdose.

In cases where the patient is uncooperative or extremely frightened, rapid tranquilization may become necessary. This process is familiar to emergency physicians, but it should be conducted with careful attention to the patient's safety, the potential risks involved, and the pharmacological characteristics of available drugs.

General Principles of Rapid Tranquilization

The following guidelines are essential for effective and safe tranquilization:

First-Line Agents: Sedative benzodiazepines and/or antipsychotics should be the preferred medications.

Oral Dosing: When feasible, oral medications are the least distressing for both patients and staff.

Familiarity with Medications: Treating physicians should be well-acquainted with the medications they administer, including knowledge of maximum safe doses and potential side effects.

Desired Outcome: The goal is to achieve a calm, cooperative patient, avoiding sedation to the point of losing airway protection, which poses significant risks.

Calm Environment: Sedated patients should be placed in a quiet, calm, and softly lit environment whenever possible.

Monitoring: Sedated patients should be monitored regularly, with a 12-lead ECG recommended for those receiving repeated doses of antipsychotic medications.

Supportive Care: Hydration, pressure care, and other supportive measures, such as deep vein thrombosis (DVT) prophylaxis, are important, especially in crowded ED settings or when patients are kept for prolonged periods.

Patient Dignity: Ensuring patient privacy by using single rooms and limiting exposure to the public is a fundamental aspect of patient care.

Risks of Rapid Tranquilization

While rapid tranquilization can be essential, it carries inherent risks, including the potential for patient or staff injury. If physical restraint is required to administer medication, it should only be performed by adequately trained staff, with mechanical restraint (such as padded straps) used in the early stages if necessary. However, restraint should not be maintained without sedation due to the risks of injury, rhabdomyolysis, and ethical concerns.

There are several known risks associated with the pharmacological management of aroused patients:

Over-sedation: Can lead to respiratory depression and pulmonary aspiration, though these are largely avoidable with proper monitoring.

Cardiac Risks: Sudden cardiac death, although rare, is a severe complication, particularly with medications that prolong the QT interval, such as thioridazine and clozapine. These medications can trigger torsades de pointes and ventricular tachycardia (VT). The risk of cardiac complications is heightened in patients with pre-existing heart conditions or conduction abnormalities.

Hypotension: Can occur with agents that have alpha-blocking effects, particularly chlorpromazine when administered intravenously.

Dystonic Reactions: Can be observed with most antipsychotics, especially with butyrophenones like haloperidol.

Neuroleptic Malignant Syndrome (NMS): A potential risk with any antipsychotic, even after a single dose.

Anticholinergic Effects: Such as delirium and urinary retention, which occur at higher doses, particularly with antipsychotics.

Seizures: Most antipsychotics can lower the seizure threshold, and benzodiazepines, especially diazepam, can accumulate and cause delirium if used repeatedly.

Elderly patients are particularly vulnerable to adverse drug reactions due to reduced hepatic metabolism and renal function, which can lead to prolonged drug effects. Even small doses of benzodiazepines can cause significant respiratory depression in this group. Furthermore, standard doses of antipsychotics can result in prolonged extrapyramidal side effects, such as mobility impairment, for days to weeks.

Pharmacological Agents

Benzodiazepines

Midazolam: A water-soluble benzodiazepine with a rapid onset of action (2 to 5 minutes via IM or IV) and a half-life of 1 to 3 hours. It is preferred over diazepam due to fewer site reactions and the ability to administer it intramuscularly. Its major adverse effect is respiratory depression, and its elimination is significantly prolonged in elderly patients.

Diazepam: Available orally or intravenously, but not recommended for IM use due to unpredictable absorption. It has a biphasic elimination, with a prolonged terminal half-life of up to 20 hours. The elderly experience prolonged effects, and it carries a risk of respiratory depression and delirium.

Clonazepam: Used orally, IV, or IM, with a prolonged elimination half-life (20 to 50 hours). Adverse effects include excessive sedation and accumulation, and it can be used for prolonged sedation.

Lorazepam: Available orally or intramuscularly, lorazepam is well absorbed and has a half-life of 12 to 15 hours. It is less likely to accumulate compared to diazepam or clonazepam and has less severe adverse effects, although excessive sedation is still a concern.

Antipsychotics

Droperidol: A potent sedative with effects seen within 3 to 10 minutes of administration, with a half-life of about 2 hours. It is also effective as an antiemetic. While controversial, the risk of cardiovascular events is not significantly higher than with haloperidol. It can cause QT prolongation, but torsades de pointes is rare.

Haloperidol: Available orally, IM, or IV, with effects peaking 20 minutes after IM injection. Its long half-life (20 hours) increases the risk of extrapyramidal effects and QT prolongation. It can also cause neuroleptic malignant syndrome.

Olanzapine: An atypical antipsychotic with a half-life of approximately 33 hours, olanzapine is effective orally or via IM injection. While it can cause sedation and mild anticholinergic effects, it is associated with a lower risk of extrapyramidal side effects and QT prolongation.

Risperidone: Available for oral and sublingual use, with a half-life ranging from 3 to 17 hours, depending on metabolism. Its adverse effects include postural hypotension and, less commonly, extrapyramidal symptoms.

These medications must be carefully selected based on the individual patient's needs, considering their medical history, age, and potential for adverse effects. Proper monitoring and ongoing care are essential to minimize risks and ensure patient safety during sedation and tranquilization.

References

1. Cong, M.L., Gynther, B., Hunter, E., & Schuller, P. (2012). Ketamine sedation for patients with acute agitation and psychiatric conditions requiring aeromedical transport. Emerg Med J, 29(4), 335–337.

2. Scheppe, K.A., Braghiroli, J., Shalaby, M., & Chait, R. (2014). The prehospital use of ketamine to sedate agitated and violent patients. West J Emerg Med, 15, 736–741.

3. McAllister-Williams, R.H., & Ferrier, I.N. (2002). Rapid tranquilization: Reevaluating the options for parenteral therapy. Br J Psychiatr, 180, 485–489.

4. MacPherson, R., Dix, R., & Morgan, S. (2005). Expanding evidence for treatment protocols. Adv Psychiatr Treat, 11, 404–415.

5. Battaglia, J., Moss, S., & Rush, J. (1997). Haloperidol, lorazepam, or both for psychotic agitation? A multicenter, double-blind study in emergency departments. Am J Emerg Med, 15, 335–340.

6. Atakan, Z., & Davies, T. (1997). ABC of mental health: Managing mental health emergencies. Br Med J, 314, 1740–1742.

7. Pilowski, L.S., Ring, H., & Shine, P.J. (1992). Rapid tranquilization: Survey of emergency prescribing in psychiatric hospitals. Br J Psychiat, 160, 831–835.

8. Alexander, J., Tharyan, P., & Adams, C. (2004). Rapid tranquilization in psychiatric emergencies: A randomized trial comparing intramuscular lorazepam and haloperidol

plus promethazine. Br J Psychiatr, 185, 63–69.

9. TREC Collaborative Group. (2003). Rapid tranquilization in psychiatric emergencies: A randomized trial of midazolam versus haloperidol plus promethazine. Br Med J, 327, 708–713.

10. Currier, G.W. (2000). Atypical antipsychotics in psychiatric emergency settings. J Clin Psychiatry, 61(Suppl 14), 21–26.

11. Department of Pharmacy. (2006). Managing agitation in older patients. Fremantle Hosp Hlth Serv Drug Bull, 30, 2.

12. Chan, E.W., Taylor, D.M., & Knott, J.C. (2013). Droperidol or olanzapine as adjuncts to midazolam in treating acute agitation: A multicenter, double-blind, placebo-controlled trial. Ann Emerg Med, 61, 72–81.

13. Calver, L., Page, C.B., Downes, M.A., et al. (2015). Evaluating the safety and effectiveness of droperidol in sedation of acute behavioral disturbances in the emergency department. Ann Emerg Med, 66(3), 230–238.

14. Wilson, M.P., Pepper, D., & Currier, G.W. (2012). Psychopharmacology of agitation: Consensus statement from the American Association for Emergency Psychiatry Project BETA Psychopharmacology Workgroup. West J Emerg Med, 13, 26–34.

15. Isbister, G.K., Calver, L.A., & Page, C.B. (2010). A randomized controlled trial comparing intramuscular droperidol versus midazolam for acute behavioral disturbance: The DORM study. Ann Emerg Med, 56, 3.

www.ingramcontent.com/pod-product-compliance
Lightning Source LLC
Chambersburg PA
CBHW071024240526
45469CB00006BD/2078